# SUPERVISION

# AND RELATED ISSUES:

## a handbook for professionals

Cathy A. Malchiodi, MA, A.T.R., LPAT, LPCC
Shirley Riley, MA, MFCT, A.T.R.

# SUPERVISION

## AND RELATED ISSUES:

### a handbook for professionals

Magnolia Street Publishers

*Published by*
**Magnolia Street Publishers**
1250 West Victoria St.
Chicago, IL 60660

ISBN: 0-9613309-7-X
Library of Congress Catalog Card Number: 96-075302
Cover Design: Sarah Reinken

Printed in the United States of America
2  3  4  5  6  7  8  9  10

# CONTENTS

# ACKNOWLEDGMENTS

First and foremost, I want to thank my many colleagues in the field of art therapy whose ideas, thoughts, and advice have helped to advance my own thinking and writing. Their generous sharing and guidance have enhanced my work as a teacher, therapist, supervisor, and author, in addition to providing both mentorship and friendship.

This book would not be possible without my many students and supervisees in art therapy, counseling psychology, social work, and other healthcare fields whose experiences have stimulated my thinking about supervision and professional issues over the last 16 years. In particular, I have learned a great deal from my students at California State University/Sacramento, Lesley College, and Southwestern College. They have helped to shape my philosophy of supervision and given me the inspiration to put my ideas on paper.

C. M.

I wish to thank the students of Loyola Marymount's marital and family art therapy program, class of 1995, for their generous contributions of drawings which illustrate the text. Their impressions of supervision and supervisory dilemmas add visual punctuation to the book.

In particular, my thanks go to the many trainees and colleagues that have shared their cases and their clinical concerns with me through the process of supervision. They have taught me, as I have taught them. Through our work together, supervision became a constant challenge to improve our understanding of the mysterious relationship called therapy.

S. R.

# INTRODUCTION

The text that follows is the work of two voices—complementary voices, I believe. We have not attempted to disguise our individual writing or intrude on each other's chapters. I am sure that the reader will notice the stylistic differences. However, we were in absolute accord as to the content of our singular contributions, which has made our collaboration such a pleasure.

Twenty years ago two women graduated from different art therapy programs...one middle aged, the other young. Over the years the two women taught, practiced in clinics and engaged in the art of supervision. In spite of very different backgrounds, we were drawn together in admiration of each other's work and found kindred spirits in the publications and presentations of the other. Our mutual respect grew as we recognized that we were philosophically in agreement about the goals of therapy. We both enjoyed helping less experienced therapists find their voices and expertise in the field of art therapy. Our attitude is what I have named an aesthetic-pragmatic approach to therapy. The therapeutic encounter contains the creative elements of artistic and imaginative solutions to difficulties while simultaneously attending to the practical solutions that give support and comfort to the client. There is a need for both ways of 'being' with our clients and our supervisees. Just as art therapy is conceptually a synthesis of two modes of communication, so should the philosophy of the practitioner embrace the dual roles of treatment.

We both also believe that it is an ethical obligation to ourselves and our supervisees to pursue our own education and keep in the forefront of our fields of knowledge. We differ in where we have concentrated our experience and continued learning. Therefore, I will now speak in my voice and let Cathy speak for herself which she does so eloquently as editor of *Art Therapy* and in her own articles and books.

I have focused my work in the field of family therapy. It is how I work and it is my belief system. I have found that successful change is more easily attained and preserved with family work. If family is not available, I still see the individual in his/her family context. I am not wedded to one theory of therapy, although I have been in love with several. I think a passionate engagement and excitement with an epistemology is the greatest joy in this work. I also think moving on to new ideas is even more stimulating. My involvement with family treatment will be noticeable in the chapters I have contributed. However, the principles of supervision do not become greatly modified when thinking about a family in contrast to thinking about an individual. The word *think* is the key to supervision. Thinking about the fundamentals of a problem, the fundamentals of treating a problem, and the fundamentals of offering the best opportunity for visual expression differs very little from thinking about the fundamentals of the belief system of the client. We all come from families of some kind, therefore it seems to be a basic experience that is common to everyone.

Supervision has been a major part of my professional life. Since 1977 I have had the privilege of being the placement coordinator for the graduate program at Loyola Marymount University, Marital and Family Therapy (Clinical Art Therapy). During that long period I supervised supervisors and students, and wrote and thought about supervision on a daily basis. However, it was not until I became immersed in this book that I realized how multifaceted the art of supervision has become. In addition to looking at clinical issues, we now must be highly sensitive to the social climate and the pressures of the mental health system. Supervision teaches the student the hard lessons of the real world. Clinical treatment and coping with the system become paramount in the supervisory relationship. It becomes progressively harder to take the first step into the world of therapeutic treatment; it is more like a plunge into the deep, armed only with newly tried skills. The novice requires support and information to make the transition from learner to therapist. Supervision is the most influential forum for learning and practicing the art of therapy. It is where theory and application of principles become real. With our supervisees we weave professionalism, creativity and human understanding into the web of treatment.

For these reasons, we must try our best to provide supervision that addresses the needs of students and novice therapists. Our supervisees must be able to provide short term therapy and crisis intervention as well as more traditionally paced therapies. We must learn to be pragmatically-aesthetic when it is called for by the situation, and then turn to an aesthetically-pragmatic approach when circumstances change. In other words, we can demonstrate that in the course of treatment the various functions of therapy have a fluid nature—both the practical needs and the creative, problem-solving needs of the client are met.

Since our supervisees will be influenced by our beliefs, we must not be rigid or inflexible as we move along in this postmodern world. However, supervision requires some form and structure. It must have a framework for ethical procedures and educational excellence. Therefore, supervision parallels the needs of the client-in-treatment and the supervisee, by focusing on case management when appropriate, and solution-focused interventions when suitable.

I hope that the text will provide an overall view of supervision and the multiple issues that impact it. It appears to be timely to offer formalized supervision guidelines that are adaptable to a variety of therapeutic settings. There are many excellent texts on supervision, but none specifically for art therapists. We hope we have started a trend that encourages the continuing development of standards and stimulates articles on supervision from other supervisors who are struggling with issues and excited about the process of supervision. There is no single answer to the challenge of supervision. Our text opens doors to exploration, raises issues, and offers ideas. We intend that readers adapt the material presented in this book and modify it to suit their own specialities and areas of interest.

Shirley Riley, 1996

As a beginning art therapist in the early 80's, I came out of graduate school with little information on how to supervise other trainees. But within a year of graduation I was expected to supervise other clinicians-in-training at my job. Soon after that I was asked to be a clinical supervisor of not only art therapy students, but also counseling psychology trainees, other creative arts therapists, social workers, and several medical students who were interested in applications of art therapy in hospital settings. At that time, I didn't stop to question my colleagues or my employer for assuming that I was skilled to supervise others; it just seemed like the natural course of events after graduation and receiving one's professional credentials.

In retrospect, although I didn't permanently maim or damage any of the unwary victims of my initial lack of expertise in supervision, I have to admit that the supervision I was able to provide in the early years was uninformed and certainly uneducated. Like many therapists, I simply was not trained to be a supervisor. However, by virtue of my graduate degree and art therapy registration I was considered to be able to supervise others. What little I had learned about supervision came from my experiences as a supervisee—from supervisors who also had no formal training in supervision.

Later, I went on to become a professor and director of two different art therapy graduate training programs, supervising student interns as part of my work. It was at that time that I began to realize the complexities of supervision and as Shirley pointed out in her introduction, the multifaceted art of supervision. I started to have many questions about supervision and began, as Shirley, to write and think about the supervisory relationship as part of my own growth and development. As I searched for information on supervision in art therapy, I also found very little published information on related topics such as how to document client progress and to prepare a case presentation, or guidelines for teaching supervisees about professional issues, ethics, or liability.

Today I think that most professionals realize that there is a great deal to be learned in order to be an effective supervisor. Despite our recognition of the complex aspects of supervision, little information has been generated on the topic and most of what is discussed is related through the oral tradition of professional conferences and educators' convocations. Some of these discussions are limited, however, with some supervisors and instructors closely guarding their methods, forms and procedures, and maybe some of their own confusion about how best to go about this relationship with trainees called supervision.

Supervision of art therapy students and postgraduate trainees is particularly challenging for many reasons. The field of art therapy, although increasing its recognition in recent years, is still evolving its identity. Supervision must be sensitive to the diversity of paths students may take to establish their identities as professionals. This may include supervision of work in clinical settings, medical milieus, community-based agencies, and even artist/therapist-in-residence situations. Because art therapy is practiced in many different settings and with disparate philosophies, supervision must take into consideration this variety and be flexible in accommodating these dimensions.

A second challenge comes from the core of art therapy itself. Since art therapists incorporate art expression as a central piece of the therapeutic process, students have unique concerns involving art products and processes to explore in supervision and training. Some of these include, but are not limited to the following: the role of art expression in treatment and assessment;

the ethics of handling and display of art expressions; and the appropriate documentation of client art. Other clinicians use art expression in therapy and assessment, but for art therapists these aspects are a principal focus, of primary interest, and a major component of successful supervision.

A third area of challenge in supervision involves the constant and erratic changes in healthcare and clinical work in recent years. In 1980 when I began my work as an art therapist, the healthcare scene was quite a different story than what it is today. Settings and ways that I practiced therapy over fifteen years ago are not applicable to today's brief therapy climate and influx of managed care. Even community-based and social service agencies where art therapists work have been impacted by these changes. In order to be of help to their supervisees, supervisors must be aware of these changes and incorporate a contemporary world view of healthcare within their supervision of trainees.

Lastly, although I believe strongly in the importance and centrality of art making as a form of therapy, self-expression, and growth, my work is informed by information from related fields. For example, in addition to my art therapy training, in recent years I have also become a licensed professional clinical counselor and am familiar with the field of counseling, just as Shirley is with marriage and family therapy. In part, this additional credential was a necessity to broaden the scope of my therapeutic work, but it has also served to give me another viewpoint of the healthcare not always available through my "profession of origin." Rather than diminishing my identity and practice as an art therapist, the infusion of this additional dimension has only enhanced my understanding of the importance of issues affecting all healthcare practitioners, including art therapists, and the realm of supervision. I hope that the reader will appreciate this additional viewpoint throughout my chapters of this text and will benefit from the perspective of a related field.

Cathy A. Malchiodi, 1996

## Some Final Notes About this Book

First and foremost, we hope that this text will serve as a practical handbook for supervisors and supervisees, as well as clinicians and instructors. We have attempted to include not only the most important topics key to successful supervision, but also the most practical areas as well.

The Table of Contents speaks for itself and we will not repeat that information in detail again here. However, we do want to highlight the major conceptual areas covered in the text. The first several chapters deal directly with issues basic to supervision, guidelines for supervision, and what to expect from the supervisory relationship, including case material and examples of difficult supervisory situations. This is followed by brief explorations of the use of the art process in supervision, peer supervision, the training and supervision of supervisors, and applications of videotape and live supervision.

The final chapters focus on issues related to supervision, including clinical writing and documentation, writing for publication, and professional and ethical issues salient to training and supervision. For the latest information on legal issues we went directly to an expert in the field of law and healthcare, Linda Randlett Kollar. Her articulate contribution to this book on the topic of legal liability is a chapter that every therapist, instructor, and supervisor should commit to memory. Linda is considered one of *the* experts in mental health law and ethics. She assists numerous therapists in this area and her experienced opinions and counsel are sought after by many healthcare professionals. We appreciate her skill, knowledge, and generosity in writing this key chapter for this text.

Lastly, we have included an extensive appendix at the end of the text. It contains a variety of actual forms and charts which supervisors may wish to copy and use with supervisees; instructors may find these useful in supervisory seminars and graduate coursework. We also have included the latest ethics document, standards of practice, and laws affecting art therapy supervision available at the time of publication. Throughout the book there are other forms as well as references and annotations to make additional supervisory materials and resources easily accessible to supervisors and instructors.

In closing this introduction, special thanks go to several people who were instrumental in helping us get this book into print. First, we would like to thank Patricia St. John, EdD, A.T.R.-BC, for reading the original draft of the text and for providing thoughtful comments and direction. Also, we would like to thank Kathryn Stern and Sarah Reinken, our publishers, for seeing this text through to its completion.

As with any first journey into uncharted territory, this effort is only a beginning. There are many other areas of supervision, training, and related issues we had to omit due to space and in the interest of giving the reader the most contemporary information available at the time of publication. However, we hope our effort has been a good beginning and that it will inspire others in our field to develop scholarly discourse and to publish theory and methodology, resulting in the deeper understanding of supervision and related issues and the continued growth of the profession.

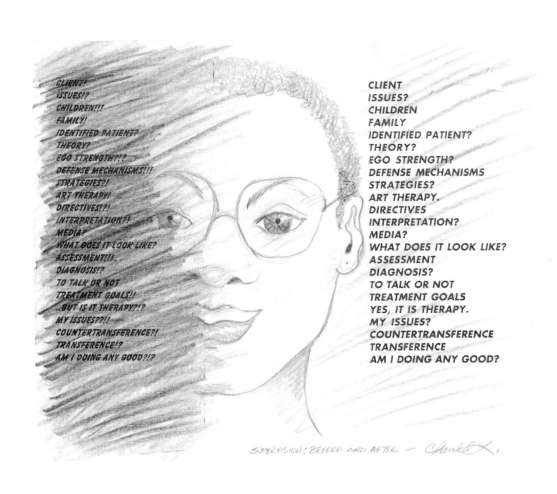

Supervision: Before and After

# CHAPTER ONE

## Art Therapy Supervision: An Overview
by Cathy A. Malchiodi

Most health-related disciplines agree that clinical supervision has recently emerged as a professional specialty (Bernard & Goodyear, 1992; Dye & Borders, 1990). However, articles, seminars, and formal supervisory training opportunities are still extremely limited, despite the fact that most healthcare professionals, including art therapists, are required to receive extensive supervision both during graduate and postgraduate training. Supervision in the training and continuing education of art therapists is considered to be essential to professionalism; this need for preparation of art therapists in supervisory skills has been noted (Wilson, Riley, & Wadeson, 1984; McNiff, 1986; Case & Dalley, 1992), but little information on the subject has been generated. How and what academic programs and placement sites teach art therapy students necessary supervisory skills is also scarce, although other allied professions have also lagged behind in this area (Ellis & Douce, 1994).

As early as 1981, the co-author of this book (Riley) initiated a series of discussion groups and panels to address art therapy supervision at the annual national conferences of the American Art Therapy Association (AATA) (Riley, 1981; Riley, Wadeson, Wilson, & Wolf, 1982). Since then those who have recognized the importance of art therapy supervision as a clinical specialty have contributed literature in the following areas: general issues of art therapy supervision (McNiff, 1986; Riley, Wadeson, Wilson, & Wolf, 1982; Wilson, Riley, & Wadeson, 1984); art therapy supervision in Great Britain (Case & Dalley, 1992; Edwards, 1993); an eclectic blend of theories and practice (Calisch,

1989); general concepts concerning the interface of art making and supervision (Durkin, Perach, Ramseyer, & Sontag, 1989; Fish, 1989); and postgraduate art therapy supervision groups (Linesch, Holmes, Morton, & Shields, 1989). However, attention to supervision and training art therapy supervisors— although a major focus of both graduate and postgraduate training— has not received much formal attention from within the field.

One reason for the lack of literature on art therapy supervision stems from the fact that materials on supervision in other disciplines already exist (see reference lists at the end of the book) and in some cases, are highly evolved (e.g. see Dye & Borders, 1990). Although this body of literature covers many of the principles common to the training of all helping professionals, it does not address the unique concerns of art therapists as supervisees and supervisors. Supervision as practiced or discussed by other clinicians may seem foreign to art therapists who are connected to the art process on both a personal and professional level. Also, those clinicians or allied professionals who use art expression in their therapeutic intervention with clients may also benefit from models of supervision that specifically include the unique element of art making within the framework. With more and more therapists using art expression in their work, supervisory and related materials that specifically address art therapy are increasingly important if clients are to be responsibly served.

Increased professionalism within the field of art therapy has also magnified the need for further articulation of both practical and theoretical aspects of supervision. Recently, the profession has moved into the area of national certification, identifying competencies and required areas of knowledge for clinical practice. In 1994, the first act licensing art therapists went into effect, including specific sections on supervision and the legal responsibilities of an art therapy supervisor (Counselor and Therapist Practice Act, 1994; see Appendix for more information). Lastly, the field of art therapy has recently updated its ethical code and standards of general and independent practice (see Appendix for more information). The content of these documents, as well as guidelines for education and training programs as put forth by the AATA, have a great impact on the need, development, and direction of art therapy supervision.

## Supervision: How Art Therapists See It

The roots of this book began with an informal survey (see Appendix A) of educators, clinicians, and supervisors to see how art therapists perceived supervision within the scope of their practices. General demographics (e.g. primary job title, number of individuals currently supervised, years as a supervisor), where supervision takes place (e.g. on site, in academic program), topics covered in supervision (e.g. case material from clients, documentation methods, ethics, legal issues, agency politics) and methods of supervision (e.g. verbal feedback/discussion, case presentation, art making ) were included in the questionnaire to examine what commonalties, if any, art therapists had in the area of supervision. In addition, several open-ended questions were included, such as "How and where did you learn to supervise?" "What are the most important issues in the supervision of art therapy students and postgraduate art therapy interns?" And, "What are the areas of art therapy supervision you would like to know more about?"

The survey sampled only a small amount of art therapists (n = 30), and was intended to generate pilot information for a larger study in the near future. However, the responses that were obtained confirmed several initial impressions that the authors had about art therapy supervision. First, its seems that most art therapists surveyed had not had any formal training in supervisory skills, stating they most often learned how to supervise from being supervised themselves, in addition to reading articles on the subject (e.g. self-study). Hence their learning was largely based on a role model or mentor during their own acquisition of clinical supervision and/or self-created through their own efforts. A few individuals had the benefit of a brief course on supervision from a graduate-level art therapy training program; the availability of such training seemed to be the exception to the rule (see Chapters 8 & 9 for a more in-depth discussion of this topic).

When responding to the question " What areas of art therapy supervision would you like to know more about?", most seemed interested in knowing more about what others were doing, how they were structuring supervision, what material they were covering in supervision, and actual techniques for supervision— in short, what a supervisor should do and what is supposed to be learned by supervisees. This reconfirmed the authors' initial impression that, on the whole, art therapists do not have a clear philosophy of supervision, the various models of how to go about supervising trainees, and the essential topics which should be covered in supervision.

## General Concepts Concerning Supervision

Holloway (1995) notes that to supervise is to "oversee, to view another's work with the eyes of the experienced clinician, the sensitive teacher, [and] the discriminating professional" (p.1). A fundamental purpose of supervision is to help trainees with their learning while at a placement and to guide their work with clients. Most professionals also observe that supervision includes helping trainees to understand their clients, developing a capacity for self-awareness and reflection, and understanding theory and practical applications of therapy to a wide range of clinical and agency settings (Dye & Borders, 1990; Hawkins, P. & Shoret, R., 1989). Supervision attempts to bring together these many different areas of learning, with the end result hopefully the development of professional identity in the trainee and the enhancement of the trainee's skills in devising successful therapeutic strategies.

In art therapy supervision, the exploration of the supervisee's feelings and reactions to clients (countertransference) has been a major focus. Mollon (1989) observed, "In supervision it is the therapy that is the patient, and the supervisee's feelings and fantasies are examined only insofar as they may throw light on what is happening in the therapy" (p.121). In a recent article on art therapy supervision, Edwards (1993) placed an emphasis on the understanding of feelings, noting the primary focus of supervision groups for art therapists are "issues, feelings and images arising from the placement situation as a whole, including the students' relationship with their placement supervisor" (p. 215). While attention to the reactions of the trainees to their clients and to supervision is important, this is a limited and simplistic view of what supervision entails. Since supervisors are legally responsible for their supervisees, supervision in the 90's goes well beyond examining transference and countertransference reactions in therapy; it encompasses ethics, laws and regulations, professional identity, and documentation, all areas of knowledge which affect the welfare and rights of clients (see Chapters 11, 12, 13, & 14 for further information). With the changes in society including cross-cultural and gender issues, violence and abuse, and reinventions of the roles of family members, supervisors must also be contemporary in their thinking about these issues which are brought to supervision. These increasingly important areas of learning are closely connected to the trainee's ability to provide interventions and services that are in the best interest of their clients.

Preparing supervisees to be part of the larger world of health professionals is considered to be central to effective supervision. Dulicai, Hays & Nolan (1989) observe three major goals in the education of arts therapists that could also be applicable to supervision:

1) learning to be a competent team member and to maintain a professional and competent identity as a therapist;

2) learning the most updated concepts in mental health and working with an increasingly widened population;

3) learning to be a competent consumer of research and to be capable of participating on a research team. (p. 11)

For trainees, learning to be part of a treatment team, along with a confidence and clarity in one's professional role, is an important developmental milestone and one which certainly should be a goal of supervision. Encouraging trainees to stay contemporary in their learning and skills is an additional concept that supervision can and should reinforce, creating a foundation for further continuing education once the formal supervisory experience has concluded. Dulicai *et al* also have noted that training in art therapy should encompass involvement with research at minimal levels of understanding, including participation as a team member, thereby strengthening trainees' recognition and respect from other professionals as well as personal competencies. Although involvement in research is a specialization that not all trainees may wish to undertake in-depth, it can be an important adjunct to clinical skills.

## Art Therapy Supervision: Is It Different from Supervision in Other Disciplines?

One of many questions that came to mind in undertaking this book was just how art therapy supervision is different from supervision in allied professions (e.g. counseling, social work, psychology, creative arts therapies)? On the surface, it is not very different in many areas of practice. There are many similarities in general treatment philosophies, ethical issues, legal matters, client welfare, that are common to all health professions. As registered, certified, and/or licensed practitioners, art therapists must abide by their own ethical code as well as the ethics and laws governing their work within the state in which they live or any additional credentials they hold. These parameters provide a framework for supervision that is similar across all health disciplines.

One major difference is obvious: the core of art therapy involves some dimension of art making and art expression. Depending on the role this plays in the art therapist's philosophy, it will have a greater or lesser effect on how s/he practices and in turn, how s/he supervises. With regard to the element of art in art therapy, some of the following unique aspects of art therapy supervision come to mind:

**1. Professional Identity:** Although most helping professions involve learning material in many divergent areas of study, synthesizing the concepts inherent to visual arts (media, processes, theory, history) and psychology (psychotherapy, counseling, marriage and family therapy ) is a unique and sometimes difficult task. Early in graduate-level training and occasionally at the postgraduate level, supervisees struggle with the question: are we psychotherapists who use art expression in intervention or are we artists who use art making as the core of therapy? Although many advanced practitioners are annoyed with this debate, it is one that becomes a problem for some trainees' and can affect their work with clients. It is also an argument that has not been resolved as yet by the profession, yet supervisors/instructors may expect students/supervisees to be able to, in a short time, develop a personal identity as an art therapist which resolves these complexities. Thus, supervision may include a focus on helping trainees produce clear definitions of the role that art plays within their work as art therapists, in addition to the identifying a theoretical framework for therapeutic work with clients.

**2. Interpersonal Skills:** In many circumstances, art therapy is still not well understood by other health professionals, clinical and agency settings. Therefore, art therapy supervision may include some extra attention to helping students or postgraduate trainees define themselves to professionals on-site through presentations and in-service trainings. Assisting supervisees in developing and honing the organizational and oral skills necessary to successful presentations to peers in related fields may be part of this task. As a secondary focus, it also may become important to recognize and discuss supervisees' frustrations in not feeling fully integrated or recognized by the facilities in which they work; the trainees' uneasiness may affect work with clients, and is therefore important to address it in supervision.

**3. Personal Philosophy:** Since there is a continuum of practice within the field of art therapy (art psychotherapy, art therapy in the schools, medical applications, more studio art-based approaches, etc.), supervision may require a special fit with supervisees' philosophies, particularly at the more advanced levels. This could be compared to trainees who are looking for clinical supervision from a strategic, a Jungian, a rational-emotive therapist, etc., but because the art process is central to art therapy, it is not exactly the same. The philosophy of how a supervisor sees the art process in the context of the therapeutic relationship is quite a different matter, and it may or may not be tied to one's particular brand of therapeutic beliefs. Since art therapy is practiced in a wide range of facilities and situations, finding a compatible supervisor who has a similar philosophy is an important component of successful supervision.

**4. Heterogeneous Learners:** Lastly, many students and supervisees come to the field of art therapy from arts backgrounds; learning has taken place in the studio, in addition to regular classroom activities. For this reason, some of the required courses which involve behavioral sciences, diagnostics, technical writing, and research may be difficult or somewhat foreign to students. Also, many students are adult learners; that is, they have returned to school in their 30's, 40's and older to obtain training and a degree. These are characteristics that supervisors may need to keep this in mind, recalling some of their own struggles and realizing that there may be many styles of learning among their supervisees.

## Types of Supervisor-Supervisee Relationships

Although it may seem like supervisory relationships are fairly clear-cut, there are a variety of possible alliances, each of which may overlap depending on the situation: 1) *Clinician-* an individual who supervises trainees usually on-site at the agency or institution at which the trainees work. S/he has direct contact with the trainee in a clinical setting, with an emphasis on clinical skill acquisition, case management, and related issues; 2) *Instructor-* an individual who supervises trainees through classroom activities. The focus of this relationship is on acquisition of conceptual and practical skills through classroom learning, but may include supervision of a clinical practicum or internship. S/he also may supervise other academic areas such as research and thesis writing; 3) *Peer-* sharing of professional experiences with colleagues. This relationship may also include an advanced supervisor who serves as leader or coordinator. Specific examples of this relationship are addressed in more detail in Chapter 7; 4) *Consultant-* an individual who supervises or provides advice on specific areas of knowledge or dimensions of treatment. Consultation may combine clinical supervision, instruction, and/or programmatic advice. It can be directed at a group of interns, students, but is more likely to be sought after by colleagues, other professionals or agencies, institutions or perhaps corporations. It most often involves the provision of specific material (e.g. art-based assessment of a family, evaluation of child abuse/neglect) and may reach into areas such as serving as an expert witness in legal matters or forensics.

These relationships are also governed by a second variable: individual versus group contact, which is the subject of the next section.

## Individual Supervision

Since most graduate training programs utilize group supervision (see below), individual supervision at the graduate level most often takes place at the practicum or internship site. The trainee may be supervised by an on-site supervisor or receive regular supervisory visits from an off-site supervisor. At the graduate level this type of supervisor may be part of a more comprehensive "learning" team that includes the site supervisor who directly oversees the trainee's clinical work; an academic instructor who sees the student in a group supervision setting or seminar and who may be the primary liaison to the site supervisor; a faculty advisor who oversees the student's entire training program and may be consulted if the student needs assistance; and possibly a coordinator of field placements who is administratively responsible for overseeing the field experience and finalizing practicum or internship agreements.

Postgraduates are more often the recipients of individual supervision, again either on- or off-site. This type of supervision is part of the trainees' continuing education as well as a necessity to meet requirements for registration, certification and/or licensure; the parameters of such supervision will be guided by the regulations governing supervision by the associations, certification, or licensing boards from whom the trainee seeks credentials. Supervision may come from professionals both within the field of art therapy and other disciplines such as psychology, social work, marriage and family counseling, and mental health counseling, depending on the trainees needs and requirements for desired credentials.

It should be noted that many art therapy students are often supervised on-site by psychologists, socials workers, counselors, or other health professionals. In the case of postgraduate supervisees, this includes supervision (i.e. 50% of the total supervisory hours) from an art therapist if the individual wishes to meet current criteria for registration with the Art Therapy Credentials Board (ATCB), and eventual art therapy licensure or certification. This art therapy supervision may be given off-site and through observation of the trainee on-site.

My personal experience as a supervisor has included students in graduate-level training programs who contract for additional supervision in specific areas of expertise outside their academic program. Although not many students can afford to do this, it is helpful to students who have a clear idea about their specific clinical or research interests. This type of individual supervision is often of a consultation nature, in which I clarify with the student exactly what types of education, guidance and training will be provided and for how long. It is always advisable to make contact with the academic program, however, to be sure there is no conflict in providing additional consultation to the student and no confusion among the student's program faculty, advisors, or other supervisors.

Lastly, art therapists may on occasion find themselves giving individual supervision to other health professionals, particularly in the form of consultation on specific topics, experiential techniques, or art expression. This is a specialized brand of supervision that involves not only the usual supervisory skills and knowledge, but also special skills and current knowledge of the use of art expression in therapeutic settings. Supervision, for example, may be in the form of evaluating and training a social worker who sees a large number of adults who were abused as children and uses drawing as a tool for communication. Although this professional may or may not be in training as an art therapist, a good supervisor (e.g. an art therapist, in this case) may be asked to provide guidance, evaluation, and consultation on the sensitive use of art expression with traumatized individuals. Or, medical personnel such pediatric nurses and child life specialists may receive art therapy supervision to better understand how their child patients view themselves, their illnesses, and medical procedures through visual art. These are a few of many examples of art therapy supervision that art therapists may provide to allied health professionals.

## Group Supervision

Group supervision is common at the graduate level of art therapy training and is prevalent in other related professions (Holloway & Johnston, 1985). It is considered to be a format for supervision which is not only economical, but also provides the added bonus of a format for peer exchange and feedback. It has some advantages over individual supervision, including peer feedback, exchange of ideas and insights, giving and receiving emotional support, and lessening dependence on the supervisor (Bratton, Landreth, & Homeyer,1993; Newman & Lovell, 1993).

There are different varieties of group supervision in art therapy, including: 1) supervisory seminars conducted by art therapy faculty within graduate level training programs; 2) supervision groups at practicum sites conducted by site supervisors; 3) postgraduate supervision groups which are designed to provide supervisory hours for registration and/or licensure; 4) peer supervision groups which may or may not have a designated leader (these are discussed in more detail in Chapter 7).

Supervisory seminars for graduate-level trainees often reflect both academic experiences and practicum/internship. They may be structured by a formal syllabus including readings, experiential work, and papers, or may be planned around a schedule of case presentations by students. Topics include any or all of the following: theoretical constructs that guide therapeutic intervention; treatment planning; participating on a treatment team; case presentation, case management, and documentation; problems/successes with clients; and ethics, laws and regulations.

Although art therapy educators and supervisors have not yet clearly defined their specific methodologies for conducting supervisory groups within graduate level training programs, they probably use one or more of the models discussed in the general literature on supervision. Holloway and Johnston (1985) have identified three major approaches used in counselor education, all of which are common to art therapy:

1.) **Interpersonal process groups:** Interpersonal process groups come from the work of Rogers (1957) when "humanistic training practices forced educators to consider trainees' affective experiences during their program of study" (p. 334, Holloway & Johnston, 1985). As a result of Roger's influence, clinical training began to embrace experiential approaches in addition to didactic methods of teaching, resulting in an emphasis on the trainees' personal exploration of clinical work.

Experiential learning is the major component of this approach; it may include direct participation, role play, dramatic enactment, and other process-oriented tasks for the purpose of learning. For example, the supervisor may ask a trainee to role play the client while the supervisor asks questions. Or, an art experiential, such as "draw your idea of an ideal client" may be used to underscore countertranference reactions. This method of learning seems like a natural approach for some art therapy supervisory groups, since experiential, self-explorative work is a foundation of art therapy training. Many art therapy supervisors at the graduate level include some form of experiential work or personal art making as part of the supervision process.

An important point to remember in using experiential work within the framework of supervision is that it does create some questions about the distinctions between therapy and training. It is likely that trainees will experience some therapeutic benefits from this type of instruction, given the personal, self-exploratory nature of this approach. Because a supervisor is also often in the role of both an evaluator of supervisees as well as a facilitator, there can be a blurring of boundaries. (Experiential approaches to supervision and related issues are discussed in more detail in Chapter 6.)

**2.) Case presentation approach:** Case presentation approaches are very familiar to art therapists and have been the staple of communication style in not only supervision, but also articles and oral presentations to other clinicians to convey clinical observations. This approach traditionally involves trainees preparing and presenting patient histories, assessment data, intervention strategies, and clinical observations concerning clients seen in the practicum or internship setting. For art therapy trainees, this includes discussion of client art expressions created in therapy.

Although case presentation has persisted in many mental health disciplines for several decades, there is little data available on this approach from any field (counseling, social work, etc.) that uses it. Art therapists may be instinctively drawn to it because it has an intuitive appeal that allows for speculation and discussion of art expressions. Although narratives about work with clients are a good thing, some format or structure is helpful to the supervisee in learning the skill of clear reporting; this skill will also be helpful in relating client material not only to art therapy peers, but also other professionals. Additional discussion of case presentation as well as documentation, is found in Chapter 11.

**3.) Developmental approaches:** Developmental theories of supervision are the most recent phenomenon of the three approaches mentioned; they involve consideration of the trainees' stage of learning in becoming therapists. These approaches may include actual instruction, group process and experiential work, and case presentation; however, the focus is on adjusting the emphasis of training according to supervisees' abilities and skills. There are various theories of stages of development in supervisees, the process of supervision and the evolution of groups; a more detail discussion of the evolution of the supervisory relationship is presented in Chapter 3.

The AATA education guidelines (AATA, 1994) recommend that group supervision at the graduate level be provided in a ratio of one supervisor to up to seven students in a group. How closely this is actually followed by programs, given restraints of money and faculty, is not known. Licensure requirements for group supervision may also differ. For example, in Massachusetts where art therapists are eligible to become licensed as clinical mental health counselors, group supervision is defined as "regularly scheduled meetings of not more than ten mental health practitioners with an approved supervisor" (Massachusetts Allied Mental Health Licensing Board, 1989). These licensure requirements, which vary from state to state, also may restrict the amount of group supervision allowable and set minimum requirements for individual supervision.

Postgraduates also receive supervision in group format. Group supervision of postgraduates may be more economical than individual; it also gives the supervisee the chance to exchange with peer professionals, in addition to the supervisor. However, as previously noted, both supervisors and supervisees should be cognizant of any regulations that restrict the inclusion of group supervision in the overall number of contact hours applicable to licensure requirements.

## Concluding Thoughts

Supervision is more than just getting together with students or supervisees on a regular basis to discuss cases and client art; many other dimensions must be considered and there are many influences on how and what type of supervision is appropriate for a specific trainee. The type of supervision may be affected by the supervisor's theoretical emphasis (systems, psychodynamic, eclectic, etc., as well as a personal theory of art therapy); a greater or lesser emphasis on explorations of feelings, countertransference, than on didactic material; requirements for case notes and presentations (including client art); preferred styles of evaluation such as video tape, audio tape and/or live supervision to evaluate the student's work; and preferred styles of teaching (through experiential, case material and/or developmental approaches).

One general rule for supervisors is to remember that although they have a responsibility to meet the training needs of the student, their primary accountability is to the clients with whom the supervisee works. Although it is often observed that supervisors and supervisees may resemble the therapist-client relationship in some sense, needless to say, a supervisor must not do therapy with a supervisee. This is not as easily separated as advocated and is an issue that must constantly be re-examined within the supervisory relationship. Cattaneo and Gawalek (1994) articulated this problem in the following way:

> "While it is common in clinical training for students to experience some therapeutic benefits from their academic work, it is incumbent on the faculty member to clarify that the clinical training is not psychotherapy. As such the student-teacher role is not a psychotherapeutic relationship - the faculty member is not in the role of therapist and the student is not in the role of a client. All core and adjunct faculty must address this issue in their course syllabus and orally discuss it with students during the introduction to the course. This is particularly important in courses which are highly experiential in nature."

Rubin (1984) makes a similar observation:

> "...it is important to remember that, if psychological problems are interfering with the supervisee's work, the answer is not becoming her therapist/supervisor; rather, it is helping her to decide on and to find a competent clinician for herself." (p.160)

Lastly, one of the most important goals of supervision is to help trainees learn to think through client cases, develop strategies to make responsible judgments about treatment, and to define ways to make the best possible decisions on their clients' behalf. Mollon (1989) observes that "the aim of supervision [is] to facilitate the trainee's capacity to think about the process of therapy..." (p.114). In the same vein, Riley (1984) notes that "supervision is the permission for the trainee to hypothesize, experiment and fantasize creative moves both with the therapeutic plan and the art expression" (p. 103). Undoubtedly, good supervision is one way to effectively clarify and improve one's therapeutic skills and to continue one's growth as a professional throughout the course of training and experience in the workplace.

## References

American Art Therapy Association, Inc. (1994). *Education standards.* Mundelein, IL: Author.

Bratton, S., Landreth, G., & Homeyer, L. (1993). An intensive three-day play therapy supervision/training model. *International Journal of Play Therapy,* 2(2), 61-79.

Calisch, A. (1989). Eclectic blending of theory in the supervision of art psychotherapists. *The Arts in Psychotherapy, 16,* 37-43.

Case, C., & Dalley, T. (1992). *The handbook of art therapy.* London: Tavistock/ Routledge.

Cattaneo, M., & Gawalek, M. (1994). *Ethical guidelines: Core and adjunct faculty multiple roles.* Cambridge, MA: Lesley College Depts. of Counseling Psychology and Expressive Therapies.

Dulicai, D., Hays, R., Nolan, P. (1989). Training the creative arts therapist: Identity with integration. *The Arts in Psychotherapy, 16,* 11-14.

Durkin,J., Perach, D., Ramseyer, J., & Sontag, E. (1989). A model for art therapy supervision enhanced through art making and journal writing. In H. Wadeson, J.Durkin, & D.Perach (Eds.), *Advances in Art Therapy* (pp. 390-431). New York: Wiley.

Dye, H. A., & Borders, L. D. (1990). Counseling supervisors: Standards for preparation and practice. *Journal of Counseling & Development, 69,* 27-32.

Edwards, D. (1989). Five years on: Further thoughts on the issue of surviving as an art therapist. In A. Gilroy & T. Dalley (Eds.), *Pictures at an Exhibition* (pp. 167-178). London: Tavistock/Routledge.

Edwards, D. (1993). Learning about feelings: The role of supervision in art therapy training. *The Arts in Psychotherapy, 20,* 213-222.

Ellis, M.V., & Douce, L.A. (1994). Group supervision of novice clinical supervisors: Eight recurring issues. *Journal of Counseling & Development, 72,* 520-525.

Fish, B. (1989). Addressing countertransference through image making. In H. Wadeson, J.Durkin, & D.Perach (Eds.), *Advances in Art Therapy* (pp. 376-389). New York: Wiley.

Holloway, E. (1995). *Clinical supervision: A systems approach.* Thousand Oaks, CA: Sage.

Holloway, E., & Johnston, R. (1985). Group supervision: Widely practiced but poorly understood. *Counselor Education & Supervision, 24,* 332-340.

Linesch, D.G., Holmes, J., Morton, M., & Shields, S.S. (1989). Postgraduate group supervision for art therapists. *Art Therapy: Journal of the American Art Therapy Association, 6* (2), 71-75.

McNiff, S. (1986). *Educating the creative arts therapist: A profile of the profession.* Springfield, IL: Charles C Thomas.

Mollon, P. (1989). Anxiety, supervision and a space for thinking: Some narcissistic perils for clinical psychologists in learning psychotherapy. *British Journal of Medical Psychology, 62,* 113-122.

Newman, J., & Lovell, M. (1993). Supervision: A description of a supervisory group for group counselors. *Counselor Education and Supervision, 33* (1), 22-31.

Riley, S. (1981). Clinical art therapy supervision. In A. DiMaria (Ed.), *Proceedings of the Twelfth Annual Conference of the American Art Therapy Association* (p. 86). Falls Church, VA: AATA.

Riley, S., Wadeson, H., Wilson, L., & Wolf, C. (1982). Art therapy supervision: theoretical considerations and administrative issues. In A. Di Maria (Ed.), *Proceedings of the Thirteenth Annual Conference of the American Art Therapy Association* (pp. 98-100). Baltimore, MD: AATA.

Rogers, C. (1957). Training individuals to engage in the therapeutic process. In C.R. Strother (Ed.), *Psychology and Mental Health* (pp. 72-96). Washington, DC: American Psychological Association.

Rubin, J. (1984). *The art of art therapy.* New York: Brunner/Mazel.

Wilson, L., Riley, S., & Wadeson, H. (1984). Art therapy supervision. *Art Therapy: Journal of the American Art Therapy Association, 1* (3), 100-105.

## Additional Readings

Biggs, D. A. (1988). A case presentation approach in clinical supervision. *Counselor Education & Supervision, 27,* 240-248.

Borders, L. D. (1991). A systematic approach to peer group supervision. *Journal of Counseling & Development, 69,* 248-252.

Holloway, E.L. (1994). Overseeing the overseer: Contextualizing training in supervision. *Journal of Counseling & Development, 72,* 526-530.

Hawkins, P. & Shoret, R. (1989). *Supervision in the helping professions.* New York:Open University Press.

Hess, A. (1980). *Psychotherapy supervision.* New York: Wiley.

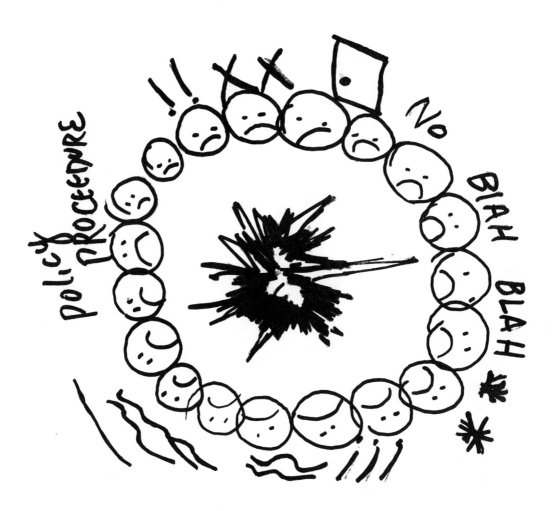

Image of a dysfunctional clinical system.

# CHAPTER TWO

## Issues Related to Art Therapy Supervision
by Shirley Riley

The task of supervision encompasses more than clinical skills and teaching therapy. Therefore, this chapter covers a variety of basic issues and concerns that impact supervision and cannot be disregarded when looking at the entire picture of supervisory responsibility. The following parallel concerns that gravely impact the success or failure of supervision will be addressed: defining the training, expertise, and specialization of the supervisor; identifying some of the restrictions that are imposed by the larger social and health system; considering multicultural issues essential to the conduct of therapy; and emphasizing the importance of continuing education. These issues will be followed by sections on the mental health workplace, the changes that have taken place recently in society, and thoughts on how to integrate services with allied professionals. The chapter concludes with a discussion of an overview of ethics and responsibilities inherent to successful supervision.

At this time, the American Art Therapy Association has not adopted standards for supervision; therefore, suggested guidelines are offered at the end of this chapter (see Table I, pg. 48). Readers are also encouraged to contact their professional associations and state licensure boards for current guidelines and standards.

### The Expertise Required of the Supervisor

To be effective, an art therapy supervisor should have at least two years of full-time clinical practice after obtaining registration. With experience, advanced supervision and continuing education, he or she will have formulated a theory of practice and developed personal stylistic strengths (Robbins, 1985).

Art therapists, at a certain point in their development, may feel personally prepared to supervise. In the profession of art therapy the decision is one that the therapist makes independently, without having to meet any criteria other than that of registration or certification. However, this is not the case in some of the allied mental health professions. For example, to be an Approved Supervisor with the American Association for Marriage and Family Therapy (AAMFT), there is a rigorous procedure that includes a course in supervision, followed by a series of documents that defend the applicant's knowledge of supervision, which is then reviewed by a committee that gives the final approval. Also, schools of social work often require a course in supervision before the licensed social worker can be a 'field instructor'. Coursework in supervision is an important component of learning to supervise because it gives the supervisor the tools and preparation needed to work with some of the problem areas noted below (see Chapter 9 for more information).

Successful supervision may require that the supervisor obtain additional training in order to help the supervisee meet his or her needs. If the supervisee is post-masters level, there may be a particular theory she or he wishes to explore. Is the supervisor willing to risk challenging some of the 'tried and true' techniques of art therapy to enhance the skills of his or her trainee? The supervisor must be responsive to the supervisee's needs and will hopefully want to integrate new thinking with concepts previously learned. The supervisor may also encourage the supervisee to reach out into the community of mental health and take some advanced courses or contact other experts in the area of interest. It would be ideal if, as part of training, supervision could include exposure to specialized seminars and conferences in allied fields of mental health. After an exposure to some new aspect of learning, discussion should take place between the members of the supervisory team; a stimulating dialogue could ensue which would only enrich supervision.

If the setting where the supervisee trains is serving a population with whom the supervisor has worked and feels competent, there is no problem. If the supervisor lacks experience with a specific population, how can this deficit in expertise be handled? Sometimes necessity forces a less than ideal situation to become the operative reality. If there are very few qualified art therapists available to supervise often a compromise must be made. This compromise should become a stimulant for the supervisor to increase his or her knowledge base. What can not be controlled must be modified in a manner that serves the population and the training team.

In some cases, supervisors are sought out because they have certain special competencies that attract the supervisee. For example, a trainee may develop an interest in working with persons of delayed development. This expertise requires specific knowledge, experience and a different tolerance for achieving goals in treatment. It is an example of specialization that takes a particular personality to achieve optimum progress with the clients in all cases. It is important that the newly trained therapist seek out not only a person proficient in the field, but also a personality that might appeal as a role model. Mentors with whom there is a high possibility of enriching ones education and encouraging ones exposure to a variety of opportunities, is a major consideration for supervision.

Lastly, the supervisor should be able to clarify the different techniques and theories that constitute individual, family, or group treatment. There are limitations and commonalties in treatment. For example; some ways of working with a family are not effective when working with an individual. However, there are similarities between family and group therapy. Perhaps the ability of the supervisor to be flexible as well as creative is truly the major task of sensitive supervision.

## Supervisory Restrictions from Healthcare Systems

There may be stipulations and stress factors imposed upon the supervisory relationship by the hospital or agency that are beyond the control of the supervisor. The supervisor may have to work with internal and external restrictions that will effect the type or form of supervision offered. Two of the limitations that must be taken into account when agreeing to supervise include:

1) If the supervisee is a graduate student, the school the student attends will have an art therapy philosophy of which the supervisor must be aware. It is confusing to the trainee to learn one theoretical approach in school and be supervised in another belief system. It is essential that the supervisor have close contact with a practicum coordinator or a faculty member and be aware of program changes and the current curriculum. Course contents evolve and the supervisor must be sensitive to, and knowledgeable of, the material that the student is learning in class (Junge,1989).

2) Is the setting a private practice, a clinic, a social service, or a hospital? In each case there will be a preferred framework for treatment: diagnostic procedures, intake forms and client history, clinical orientation, or emphasis on long or short-term treatment. Each of these procedures will be defined by the setting. If the supervisor is not familiar with the agency's formats, the supervision may be at odds with the learner's best interests.

For example, it would be uncomfortable for the supervisee to present a case in clinical conference where the treatment plan suggested in supervision was based on long-term psychodynamic theory, while the clinic or hospital had expected the intern to follow strategic short term crisis interventions. This is an exaggeration of bad judgment, but it does underscore the fact that art therapists need to join the mainstream of current eclectic therapeutic thinking in the mental health field (Nichols & Schwartz, 1995).

## Defining Art Therapy

As has often been said, art therapy does not exist in a vacuum (Calisch, 1989). Often the art therapist is asked to articulate to colleagues and extended staff team "what is art therapy?", or "what do you do with that art?" Finding an answer to these questions that is coherent and comprehensible to fellow professionals is not something that comes to the novice without careful consideration and coaching by the more experienced supervisor.

In addition to aiding new therapists in their understanding of the theoretical component of treatment, the supervisor must assist supervisees until they are able to explain, in clinical terms, the process of art therapy. With so many agencies limited to counselors, social workers and psychologists, it is particularly important for art therapists to have the skill to present their work in a manner that is understandable to allied professionals in the workplace. The ability to explain how clinical skills facilitate the art therapy treatment is often the best way of understanding the process; therefore, a cogent presentation benefits the supervisee on many levels.

## Supervision & Special Populations

Theoretical focus is a basic concern when deciding on the appropriate treatment for special populations. For example, hospitalized patients need a different form of art therapy than the ADHD child in a school program. There is always a possibility that a wrong approach will cause greater agitation in the more severely distressed client. Unless the treatment is closely tailored to the client's tolerance for new material to surface in the art, the art therapy may not be helpful. Many clients are only able to handle limited stimuli; for example, the hyperactive child may need to have an active, but contained, involvement with the art process, while the psychotic client's treatment may depend a great deal on the issue of his or her medication. Also, the impact of primitive imagery, which may surface in the art representations of the psychotic patient, must be monitored.

The supervisee must be alerted that clients may be disturbed when viewing each other's artwork. For example, in hospital groups the therapist must be constantly alert to the possibility that if one client draws images that are grossly suggestive of frightening threats, another member of the group may take in these images and decompensate. Artworks are powerful tools of expression and in a group all the art is open to be experienced by all the group members. Discretion must be used with dissociative clients who may not be ready to incorporate the visual memories that emerge in their art product (Spring, 1993; Cohen & Cox, 1995). Artwork can cause flashbacks that are not appropriate to the client's stage of recovery. In addition, the therapist working with the severely abused client must know how to protect and calm the agitated client. Other examples where discretion is necessary are too numerous to list here, but each form of caution and the capacity to shape the treatment to the needs of the special population is of primary concern in supervision.

For many art therapists working with abused children and adults, caution in the timing and pacing of the therapy must be emphasized in supervision (Levinson,1986; Malchiodi,1990). Supervision that guides the trainee to cope with abusive situations takes special research into not only the dynamics, but also the case management issues. The issues of reporting and legal demands, involve more concerns than clinical practice (see Chapters 13 & 14 on ethics and legal issues). In their practicums, interns are dealing with cases of molestation, domestic violence, and suicidal ideation (to name a few). These are problems that were assigned only to the experienced clinician in the past. Now, with reduced staff and rising violence in society, the beginner is often forced to cope beyond her or his skill. Supervision is the first place that the beleaguered intern will turn and the supervisor must be available. Encouraging trainees to seek out their peers in a support group (see Chapter 7 on peer supervision), offering extra supervision time when crisis arise, and helping the beginner not ask the impossible of themselves, can be contributions the supervisor makes to keep the supervisee from early burn-out.

To summarize, art therapy offered in hospital or day treatment differs dramatically from outpatient treatment. Art therapy in schools differs from art therapy in a wellness clinic; geriatric treatment has it's own characteristics. This list could continue for as many settings as art therapy has been utilized. In every case the supervision differs as radically as the contrasting needs of the population. The environment constantly places restrictions and incentives on the supervisory task.

## Cultural Considerations

How to work with a client of an ethnic background which differs from that of the supervisee is an issue that must be directly addressed in supervision (Jenerson, 1990). How to introduce the subject of two different cultural backgrounds and two world views into the session and how to encourage a dialogue with the client are skills that a new intern may not have learned. In most training programs multiculturalism is a required classroom subject. However, actually talking to persons about trusting you as their therapist, when you probably do not understand the pressures and truths of their culture, is quite another matter. If the supervisee is working with a person of a culture that the supervisor knows little about, then both should find resources that address the subject before misunderstandings cloud the therapy.

Jenerson (1990) suggests:

> "In order to facilitate cultural sensitivity, it is important for the supervisor to explore with the supervisee each of their particular ways of viewing the world, their ethnic identifications, their values, and the cultures. Not being aware leaves one open, placing one's personal values upon the client or the supervisee. This exploration can be done in a very positive and sharing manner as an educational aspect of the supervision. . . . Supervisees' culturally sensitive concerns, stereotypes and fears should be openly addressed so that their knowledge about cultural issues can be broadened. . .This experience cuts across all permutations of race, sex, religious orientation and social class." (p. 3-47-48)

The supervisor may suggest that an open discussion with the client will do wonders to reduce discomfort. Often a person of another background will be pleased to educate the therapist about issues that have unique meaning in their culture. If they are not willing to discuss this issue, the client has at least heard that his or her cultural meanings are valuable to the therapist. This dialogue should also encompass the metaphors and symbolic images that appear in the art (Dufrene,1991; Steinhart,1986). Some symbols may be specific to the culture and convey significance that is not recognized by the therapist.

In contrast, there are times when the supervisor and the supervisee may know a lot about their own cultures, but they do not share the same culture. This is a unique challenge that is not easy to solve completely. The positions between the two are not equal; the supervisor has more power. This imbalance may make the discussion about divergent ethnicity awkward. The supervisor must be the leader in this dialogue and bring up the differences in color, background, religious beliefs, or whatever seems appropriate to discuss about the differences in their life experiences. Denial of difference is the danger, not the dialogue.

Jenerson (1990) has an important observation:

> "What about the situation when the supervisee is a member of a people of color and the supervisor is a member of the dominant culture? Many might take the 'color blind' approach and treat the situation the same as if both were from the same dominant group without being sensitive to cultural issues. This would be a

grave error. This reversed situation presents a unique opportunity for the supervisor to learn, in close, intimate setting, more about a person of another culture." (...and an equal learning occasion for the supervisee also; authors comment) (pp. 349-350)

Finally, there is the situation where both the supervisor and supervisee are people from the same ethnic background(s). In this type of supervisor-supervisee relationship, there is an additional issue the supervisor may fail to explore cultural issues on the assumption that since the supervisee is already a person of color, he or she automatically understands and is sensitive to these issues. The reality is that both persons may still be evolving through various stages of their individual ethnic identifications.

## Continuing Education

Theories and methodologies of the last few years are radically different than those of the preceding decades. Hopefully, the supervisor reads the latest material rather than being content with old information. The supervisor should be most attentive to their prejudices; we all carry more around than we confess to! Gender issues and role assignments still plague our perceptions of each other. The challenge from feminist therapists has resulted in one of the most dramatic shifts in thinking in therapeutic theory in many years (Gilligan, 1982, 1993; McGoldrick, Anderson, & Walsh. 1989). Another major shift came with the introduction of the concepts of social constructionism (Anderson & Goolishian, 1988) and narrative conversation (White & Epston, 1990).

These considerations and more, should be areas of ongoing investigation by the supervisor. Thoughtful supervisors can encourage and enrich the knowledge of their supervisees by supporting their curiosity and reinforcing their desire to attend conferences, seminars and lectures. Acquiring continuing education may also be useful for some professional credentials. By attending classes themselves, the supervisor becomes an example of the desire to change and risk old belief systems—modeling the flexibility and commitment to growth that they desire for their supervisees.

## Social Concerns and Their Impact on Therapy & Supervision

Contemporary sociological pressures are issues of primary importance to treatment. The supervisor must use the daily newspaper and the media as additional texts to more competently guide their supervisees when evaluating the needs of the client. Diagnosing a crisis in the current socio-economic cauldron is difficult for even the most experienced clinician. Attention to the realities of our client's lives will do a great deal to de-pathologize their diagnosis.

The treatment of the clients cannot be separated from the realities of the world in which we all live. Their additional burdens, by reason of socio-economic position, skills, color, and gender must be considered. Their strengths, family systems, special knowledge, unfamiliar beliefs and religious practices, and the position of men and women in their society, must not be overlooked in the search for solutions of problems. The unfamiliar attitudes encountered in therapeutic relationships should be approached with interest and acceptance, even though they seem at variance to notions of equality, or many other 'American' standards.

This freedom to be the learner, instead of the authority, is an unfamiliar position for many new therapists. Supervisees often define their role as a 'healer' or 'creative facilitator'. It is a gift from the supervisor to help them into their new role as the student of their client's ways.

## The Workplace

Therapists who practiced therapy in the late 70's and 80's are saddened when they see work conditions that have a negative impact on their supervisees. Economic pressures on the facilities deprive the trainee of many of the necessary support systems expected for the new therapist. On-site supervision is one of the essentials that fall into this category. It is infinitely better to supervise on-site than off-site; the on-site supervisor is available for brief moments for advice and support. The on-site supervisor also appreciates the internal politics of the workplace and can screen the cases that are assigned to the trainee.

Politics are not usually considered when selecting a training site. However, politics greatly influence the supervisee's performance. When the structure in which you work is in crisis, then that crisis reverberates throughout the system. We are powerless to change the larger system, but neither do we have to take an over humble position that denies us an equal share of whatever resources are available in the community.

It is important that the off-site supervisor be recognized by the facility where the trainee is in practicum, or where the intern is employed. For example, the supervisor could offer an in-service for the general staff and in this manner educate the agency about art therapy and introduce the trainee as a clinical member of the team. Often the art therapist is out numbered by the other professionals and her or his role not well understood by the staff. The supervisor can make a difference in the staff's perceptions by showing expertise and clinical knowledge; this will favorably reflect on the supervisee.

One of the most common complaints and the situation most uncomfortable for the novice art therapist to handle, is the requests from the staff to "tell us what this kid's drawing means." The art therapist feels that it is threatening to their position and bordering on unethical, to share techniques of art therapy, unless they can convey full knowledge of the principles of treatment with visual expression. Since this is not possible, a little information can be offered by way of referring the staff person to a basic text on art therapy. However, if the supervisor can present an in-service to the staff, she or he can circumvent this dilemma by the education offered through a case conference or seminar.

## The Mental Health Situation: Year 2000

The new art therapist is entering the marketplace at a time of uncertainty of the status of healthcare. With changing attitudes regarding health care and the introduction of managed care, unpredictability is bound to have an impact on a therapist's development. It is hard to focus on techniques and theories when one's head is full of doubts about the job market and paying back a student loan.

Supervisors must be as attentive to the reality of the supervisees' world, just as they caution them to be sensitive to the reality of the client's world. The palmy days of mental health funding are over and supervisors should not only help supervisees clinically, but also keep them in touch with any new developments in the general service providers domain. For example, an issue of the *Family Therapy Networker* devoted attention to the necessity of the practitioner bringing a variety of skills to the field of mental health that therapists have ordinarily tried to avoid. A practice consultant (Lawless, 1995) is quoted:

> "Many therapists are great clinicians, but terrible business people, temperamental people in a profession that is changing from being an art to an industry. These changes cause a lot of cognitive dissonance. ...some clinicians can make the change and learn to explain themselves to the business community...but for others altering themselves to fit the pattern of consumer capitalism cuts too close to the marrow of their personal identity. Some even leave the field rather than make these compromises."(p.24)

How to network and negotiate the job market does not seem a traditional skill required of a supervisor. However, if this is the dominant concern of the supervisee, it has to be addressed and put in perspective. Some suggestions to the supervisee could be: joining local professional associations and other organizations in allied fields; networking with colleagues; presenting case studies to interested groups in the community; and appling for jobs that ask for mental health professionals, but not necessarily art therapists. None of these ideas are particularly original, but the attention to the new therapist's anxiety will support their creative attack on the system and give them understanding at this difficult time.

In today's healthcare climate the danger of being sued is high and it is an ethical issue to be covered. The supervisor should also make sure that the supervisee carries malpractice insurance. The professional organizations have brochures and information available to supply on request. The higher levels of tension in society have raised the percentage of legal suits and the beginning practitioner must be protected. Of equal importance is adequate malpractice insurance for the supervisor. He or she is in an exposed position to be sued if the supervisee is breaking the law or the ethical standards of the profession. It is important to be sure the insurance has an adequately high monetary coverage. If the supervisor has a license, he or she should carry insurance that covers it.

## Encouraging Integration with Allied Professionals

Art therapists are not separate from other therapeutic disciplines. All therapists share the responsibility and the hope that they will offer persons in distress an opportunity to achieve the change they desire. They use their skills in the service of their clients and in conjunction with other professionals in the mental health world. It is a mistake to emphasize our differences at the expense of being a valid and powerful member of the team. The art therapist's identity, that some seem to feel is so fragile, will be a non-issue if the profession is not integrated into the general health services. Supervisors and their supervisees are essential in the formation of a strong identity and purpose within healthcare that insure the continued growth of the profession.

National art therapy conferences have invited professionals from other fields to present at yearly meetings. It is equally important that art therapists present at other conferences outside their specialty, and supervisors should encourage supervisees to do so. Cross-fertilization is one answer to recognition and continued survival in the job market.

## Personal Ethics, Responsibilities, and Commitments

A question concerning supervision remains: Are all registered or board certified art therapists qualified to supervise? The answer to this question is the personal and ethical responsibility of each individual. It ultimately is one which must be confronted by each person who chooses to supervise. There are no restrictions at this time in regard to becoming a supervisor. Just because we have a credential that says we have professional permission to supervise, do we have the requisite personality, training, desire, and curiosity to improve our knowledge base that the role of supervisor demands? Therefore, the answer lies in a self-search, an activity questioned by no one but the individual themself.

In Chapter 3, the importance of the supervisory relationship is identified as the most significant transforming and educational portion of a new therapist's growth. However, in the art therapy profession, the guide on this journey of learning is a person that has rarely had specific training as a leader or has had to prove that he or she has any particular talents to assume this position of mentorship or teaching. Until training and evaluation in supervision is established, therapists are burdened with the decision of their own worth in this role of supervisor.

Not everyone is capable of teaching or supervising. Stieny (1995), speaks from her extensive experience teaching supervision and being a supervisor:

> "Some therapists are adequate clinicians but operate from such a instinctual base that they cannot, indeed, prefer not, to 'destroy' their spontaneity with theoretical explanations. Others are deeply involved in appreciating visual expression, but are tongue tied when they try to express themselves in words. None of these traits, and others in a similar vein, necessarily make a less competent therapist, in the right setting, but it does not help with teaching. The greater question is; Is it even possible for us to learn to modify our disposition?" (p.2)

Some personalities are hypersensitive to other person's reactions or actions, shy, or find expressing their opinions difficult for fear they may be misinterpreted. If this is the person's dominant reaction, how can he or she be a supervisor and offer or confront difficult corrective criticism that may be necessary? If we are in a transitional period of our life where personal circumstances are particularly critical and thought-consuming, can we admit to ourselves that we have insufficient resources to share in the *giving* relationship of supervisor at this time? Finally, is the supervisor-to-be willing to continue her or his own education? Does he or she accept that only with self growth can one person be a model for another person's growth? Is the possibility of continuing in personal therapy a matter that is reflected upon, or, if not therapy, perhaps a peer group for consultation and clinical challenge?

What is really being asked is the moot question: have we taken the time to deeply explore what this commitment to supervision means? Not everyone is suited for the supervisory role. It entails legal and ethical responsibility and a commitment of time that often has a low monetary return, or perhaps none. For example, when a conflicting financial opportunity arises, do you feel the first responsibility still remains with the supervisory relationship until the training contract has expired?

Can we become more sensitive to our own bias and reactive behaviors? What is the stance we have taken in regard to gender issues? Gender assigned roles? There are political and personal topics (e.g. abortion) which are exceedingly emotional questions for many persons, but still have to be dealt with in the clinical and supervisory session with neutrality and distance. Will that be a problem for the supervisor? Do we believe that therapy is a forum for an activist stance? How can we protect the victim and still have understanding for the abuser? Can anyone really be neutral in highly charged abusive situations? What counsel can you give yourself in these dilemmas that have no clear answers and speak to the very foundations of a world view? In the final analysis, you must be the one to decide if you are temperamentally suited to teach and mentor within the format of supervision.

## Conclusion

This chapter has covered a wide range of related issues that have an impact on supervision. What has emerged as the central theme is the recognition that supervision is not just a clinical or educational relationship, but is a composite of many factors emanating from society and the healthcare system. The skills of the supervisor are modified by the systemic restrictions that may be placed upon that supervisor. How those restrictions are incorporated into the supervisee's training is an important factor. The ability of the trainee to explain in clear clinical terminology the advantages and theories of art therapy treatment is an additional aspect of coaching that enriches the supervisor's role. Looking at the very important issues of the needs of special populations, as well as the cultural considerations between client and therapist and supervisor and supervisee, cannot be over emphasized. Where we practice and under what conditions of support, comfort, or political pressure are issues that must be considered. How the supervisor incorporates all of these issues, as well as help the intern to integrate theories of allied professions with his/her own belief system, demonstrates the role modeling that is an important component of supervision. We are a part of the post modern world and how we think about art therapy supervision should take a progressive stance. Future standards for supervision will provide a base from which to grow and find improved ways to cope with the changing world of mental health.

## References

Anderson, H. & Goolishian, H. (1988). Human systems as linguistic systems: Preliminary and evolving ideas about the implications for clinical theory. *Family Process, 27,* 371-394.

Calish, A. (1989). Eclectic blending of theory in the supervision of art psychotherapists. *The Arts in Psychotherapy, 16,* 37-43.

Cohen, B. & Cox, C. (1995). *Telling without talking.* New York: W.W. Norton.

Cohen-Lieberman, M.S. (1994). The art therapist as expert witness in child sexual abuse. *Art Therapy; The Journal of the American Art Therapy Association, 11*(4) 260-265.

Cox, L. (1990). Integrative evaluations: Some processed oriented questions for supervisors. In *Practical Applications in Supervision* (pp.85-90). San Diego: CAMFT.

Dufrene, P. (1991). Comparison of treatment of traditional education of native American healers with education of American art therapists. *Art Therapy; Journal of the American Art Therapy Association, 8*(1), 17-22.

Gilligan,C. (1982). *In a different voice.* Cambridge, MA: Harvard University Press.

Goldenthal, P. (1993). A matter of balance: Challenging and supporting supervisees. *The Supervision Bulletin* (AAMFT), 3 (2), 1-2.

Hines, M. (1993). In my opinion: Dual aspects of dual relationships. *The Supervision Bulletin* (AAMFT), 6 (3), 3.

Junge, M. (1989). Co-perspective: The heart of the matter. *The Arts in Psychotherapy, 16* (2), 77-78.

Jenerson, D. S. (1990). Practical and cultural aspects of supervision. In *Practical Applications in Supervision* (pp. 43-51). San Diego:CAMFT.

Lawless, M. (1995). *The Family Therapy Networker*, Vol. 19, #4, p. 24.

Levinson, P. (1986). Identification of child abuse in art and play products of pediatric burn patients. *Art Therapy; Journal of the American Art Therapy Association, 3* (2).

Malchiodi, C. (1990). *Breaking the silence: Art therapy with children from violent homes.* New York: Brunner/Mazel.

McGoldrick,M.,Anderson,C., & Walsh,F. (1989). *Women in families: A framework for family therapy.* New York: W.W.Norton.

Nichols, M.P., & Schwartz, R.C. (1995). *Family therapy: Concepts and methods.* Boston, MA: Boston, Allyn and Bacon.

Robbins, A. (1988). A psychoaesthetic perspective on creative arts therapy and training. *The Arts in Psychotherapy, 15* (4),95-100.

Schwartz, R. C. (1995) *Internal family systems therapy.* New York: Guilford Press.

Spring, D. (1993). *Shattered images: Phenomonological language of sexual trauma.* Chicago, IL: Magnolia Street Publishers.

Steinhart, L. (1986). Art therapy in Israel. *Art Therapy: Journal of the American Art Therapy Association, 1* (3), 3-6.

Steiny, N. (1995). Editorial. *Newsletter: California Association of Marriage & Family Therapists,* 1, 2.

White, M. & Epston, D. (1990). *Narrative means to therapeutic ends.* New York: W.W. Norton & Co.

## TABLE I

## Suggested Guidelines for Art Therapy Supervision
### Shirley Riley & Cathy A. Malchiodi

Supervision of art therapists is a distinct field of preparation and practice. The following suggested guidelines describe the training, knowledge, and competencies that characterize effective art therapy supervisors.

## I. Supervisor Qualifications
### A. General:

A supervisor shall have been a Registered Art Therapist (A.T.R.) for at least two years prior to acting as a supervisor; will not be under censure for any ethical malfeasance; and should not be related by blood or marriage to the supervisee or have a personal relationship with the same that may undermine the effectiveness of the supervision.

### B. Training:

A supervisor will have a graduate degree and training that includes the core curriculum and practicum hours suggested in the AATA Education Standards (AATA, 1994). In addition, the supervisor will have a current credential plus two additional years of active practice and is currently an active clinician. The supervisor will have had post-graduate training in supervision including courses/seminars.

### C. Experience:

A supervisor will have had supervised experience in an approved agency that provides health care to the public. The supervisor will have trained for at least one year in an institution serving a population similar to that of the supervisee's current placement/employment. The supervisor will also have a broad understanding and education in art therapy theory and practice that is compatible with the supervisee's current placement/employment.

### D. Additional Qualifications:

The supervisor demonstrates a knowledge of differences with regard to gender, race, ethnicity, culture, and age, understanding the importance of these characteristics in clients and in the supervisory relationship; is sensitive to the evaluative nature of supervision; understands the developmental nature of supervision and uses supervisory methods and materials appropriate to the supervisee's level of conceptual development, training and experience; can identify learning needs of supervisee and adjusts consultation to best meet these needs.

## II. Continuing Education

Continuing education is recommended for all supervisors. The focus of the continuing education courses should be on improving skills in supervision and evaluation and should assist the supervisor in acquiring additional knowledge of theory and practice in which supervisees are training.

## III. Responsibilities of Supervisors

### A. General:

The supervisor will be responsible for the extent, type, and quality of the art therapy performed by the supervisee. Supervisors will be compliant with all laws, rules and regulations governing the practice of art therapy with clients and consumers: knowledge of AATA ethical codes and related codes of ethics; regulatory documents that impact the profession (certification, licensure, standards of practice, etc.); knowledge of ethical considerations that pertain to the supervisory relationship (dual relationships, evaluation, due process, confidentiality, and vicarious liability).

### B. Knowledge of Supervisory Methods & Techniques:

The supervisor:

• is clear about the purpose of supervision and the methods to be used;

• works with the supervisee to decide direction of supervisory experiences;

• uses appropriate supervisory interventions such as art tasks, role-play, modeling, live supervision, homework, suggestions and advice, review of audio and video tapes;

• makes every effort to observe the supervisee in the practice of art therapy with clients (e.g. audiotape, videotape, or live supervision);

• uses media to enhance learning (printed material, tapes, art process);

• understands how to facilitate the supervisor's self-exploration and problem-solving;

• devises a method of evaluation which will inform the person being supervised of the quality of his/her clinical abilities and learning experience;

• can serve as an evaluator and can identify the supervisee's professional and personal strengths as well as weaknesses.

### C. Case Management

The supervisor:

• recognizes that the primary focus of supervision is the client of the supervisee;

• assists the supervisee in choosing assessment procedures and interventions;

• assists in planning therapy and prioritizing client goals and objectives;

• assists the supervisee in providing rationale for art therapy interventions;

• assists with the referral process, when appropriate;

• assists the supervisee in effectively documenting interactions with clients and identifying appropriate material to include in verbal or written reports;

• assists the supervisee in areas of confidentiality of client and supervisory records;

• is cognizant of the roles of other professionals at the supervisee's placement/employment;

• requires the supervisee to keep an accurate record of client contact and signs these records monthly.

## IV. Other:

1. Supervision is conducted in a ratio of one hour of supervision to every ten hours of the supervisee's client contact, or as required by certifying agencies and/or licensure boards. Graduate-level trainees' supervision also conforms to any additional program requirements of the educational program.

2. Supervision is a confidential contract between supervisor and supervisee. Both the supervisee and the supervisor will not breach client confidentiality unless there is a question of danger to the client or unethical performance on the part of the trainee.

3. The supervisor will advise the supervisee that all client artwork is part of confidential clinical records. If client artwork is to be utilized for display or reproduced for clinical or educational presentations, a written release must be obtained from the client. Any identifying marks should be disguised or removed prior to presentation or display.

4. If the supervisor has concerns about the ability of the supervisee to do art therapy, it is the supervisor's responsibility to share these concerns with the supervisee. The supervisor should decide how to best help the supervisee, and, if this is not possible, the supervisor will not sign for hours and will terminate supervision. The supervisor should encourage the trainee to acquire additional training before resuming work as an art therapist with clients.

---

*Readers are again reminded that these guidelines are offered as suggested standards only. Please contact the AATA, ATCB, and/or other professional organizations and licensure boards for current standards of practice regarding supervision.*

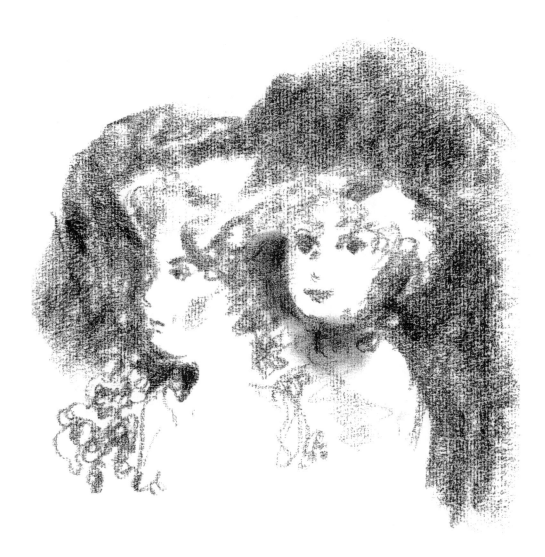

Supervision: I feel when I relate the events of a session, my supervisor has the ability to re-experience the session. Her uncanny sense of what went on allows her to offer me an accurate direction in which to work with clients... I also feel as if she is there with me as her words blend with mine—shaping, giving strength and form to our work.

# CHAPTER THREE

## The Evolution of the Supervisory Relationship
by Shirley Riley

This chapter examines the multi-level aspects of the supervisory relationship. A variety of issues will be examined: the techniques of supervision; the structural and contractural considerations; personal anxieties of the novice therapist; and personality conflicts between supervisee and supervisor. The developmental approach will be emphasized by considering the process of maturation reflected by the ability of the supervisee to conduct therapy and to appreciate the central position of the art in the therapy. Finally, the question of maturity, both with the supervisee and supervisor, will be examined.

Often supervision has been described in developmental terms (Ard, 1973; Cohen, Gross, Turner,1976; Everett, 1981; Friedman & Kaslow, 1986; Hess, 1986 and as a teaching-through-modeling opportunity (Liddle & Saba, 1982; Schwartz, 1988). Supervision constitutes the most important clinical and educational experience in a new therapist's training (Kaslow, 1984). The linear progression through stages of development is only one aspect of this complicated relationship. Many issues arise in supervision, including: 1) the educational aspect; 2) the intrapersonal actions between supervisor and supervisee; 3) the impact of the larger systems of the workplace; 4) the power of social factors on both the trainer and the trainee; and 5) the legal and ethical considerations that are ever-present in the therapeutic contract.

### Parallel Process

Not only are there linear developments, but even larger systemic, circular interactions which must be addressed. Supervisors are ultimately responsible for the therapy conducted by their supervisees, both ethically and legally, and must be concerned not only with the experience of the supervisee but the client as well. There is often the struggle to successfully convey information from client through supervisee to supervisor and then to reverse the process. The parallel process (Ekstein & Wallerstein, 1972) is a powerful component of the supervisory procedure:

> "Should we therefore wonder at the surprise of so many a beginning therapist, selecting the patient's material, distilling it through the vehicle of the emphases dictated by his own needs, and presenting it thus to the supervisor, when he discovers what he sees and presents often so closely parallels comparable problems he himself experiences in supervision. Whether it be of beginning, of termination, or of process in between, therapist and patient seem to be constantly working on the same problems. Only as the student is helped in the resolution of such difficulties in himself, will he or she be able to objectively see the enlarged aspects of the patient's problems. It is though we work with a constant "metaphor" in which the patient's problem in psychotherapy may be used to express the therapist's problem in supervision—and vice versa." (p.179-180)

This parallel process in supervision reflects the relationship between client and therapist and between supervisee (therapist) and supervisor and, therefore between supervisor and client through the supervisee. How the supervision is experienced by both professionals is enacted upon the client(s). The process is also complicated by conscious and unconscious factors.

Emotions are stirred up in both parties while guiding the client's therapy. The subsequent transference of these emotions to the relationship between the supervisor and trainee may bring attention to personal sensitive areas. The principle of parallel process is "a change in any aspect of the supervisory relationship that is reflected throughout the levels of the therapeutic system"(Doehrman, 1976).

The complexities of supervision are as broad as the involvement in a therapeutic relationship. Gillen (1990), discusses the issue of counter-transference:

> "In order to use diagnostic countertransference, interns need to be able to differentiate between feelings that come from their own past and those that are generated by others. The interns should have enough observing ego to be able to make this distinction. The only way it is possible for interns to develop a clear enough observing ego is to have worked through their own historical material to the degree they understand how it may influence their involvement in the client's therapy. When they are sufficiently familiar with family of origin material and its effects, they have attenuated the emotional charge enough, that when it is triggered they can stay in contact, both with their own material and with their clients." (p. 158)

## Examining the Process of Treatment

The supervisor is obliged to reveal how she or he arrived at the clinical conclusions under discussion in supervision. Revealing the decision-making process that led to an intervention does not offer the safe, anonymous stance that some supervisors choose to use in the client/therapist situation. The honest sharing of doubts, indecisions and fortuitous moves made during the session are educational for the intern to hear. It allows the trainee an opportunity to enter into the decision-making process of the more experienced clinician. If the decisions made in supervision for the conduct of the client's therapy are not highly successful, the clients might not challenge the therapist. In contrast, the supervisee should be encouraged to challenge their supervisor's decisions. As therapy progresses, changes made in the session often are not recognized. They are more clearly revealed through close examination at a later date in supervision. It is an old axiom that working through a mistake produces the greatest opportunity for mutual learning to take place. However, admitting to errors becomes more difficult when one's professional image is at stake.

In order to make some sense of all these intricacies I propose to look at the issues of supervision and am aware that they rarely present themselves in order and vary dramatically with each supervisee.

## Contractual Issues

The first contact between supervisor and supervisee must be one that clearly delineates the structure of how they will proceed. The time and length of the supervision is established. The conditions concerning changed or cancelled appointments and financial charges are written into this contract. Negotiations around these issues are handled in the first session, including the possibility of clinical emergencies and who will cover the crises. Clarity at this early moment will protect both parties from distress in the future.

In California there are Laws and Regulations concerning supervision which are delineated in the *California Association of Marriage and Family Manual; Practical Applications in Supervision* (CAMFT ,1990). These rules may not be applicable to other regions of the country, however, it is a good model to review. They clearly state the requirements regarding hours of supervision per client, the number of persons in a supervision group and many other issues that have to do with the structure and accountability that is expected from the supervisory relationship. Social workers, psychologists and counselors each have specific guidelines that provide information to their profession regarding supervision.

Another contractual issue concerns the form and frequency of progress notes or case write-ups. Supervisors must discuss requirements for recordings of the supervised sessions including the form, the length, and how the presentation of the art work will be incorporated in the case review. The supervisee is responsible for coming prepared with this material to the supervisory appointment. Procedural questions and the format of the hour are to be thought through with care prior to the appointment. Time spent on these structural details will help free both members of this association from tensions and misunderstandings later on. Like a good marriage contract, the expectations should be explicit, not implicit (Sluzki, 1974).

The supervisor should be prepared to discuss her or his qualifications, training and philosophical belief system concerning the practice of therapy. Goldenberg and Goldenberg (1991) discuss the need for the family-oriented therapists to define their position versus the individually-oriented therapists. Their discussion highlights the need for a dialogue with trainees concerning the philosophy of the supervisor. Supervisees should feel confident that they are getting the best possible training available and that their supervisors are experienced and qualified to work with the patient population they will be presenting in supervision. An environment is established that provides the security to encourage the beginner to ask questions and the assurance that confidentiality will be maintained if personal issues surface in the course of supervision. Kaslow (1986) states:

> "...supervisors and trainers and their trainee counterparts are likely to gravitate toward that methodology (ies) which is (are) most compatible with their own philosophy, personality and style. If pressured into utilizing or submitting to an approach that is ego dystonic, it is likely not to prove viable for a specific supervisor or supervisee; conceivably he or she will in some way sabotage its effectiveness in order to demonstrate its unworkability so as to be free to utilize a process, model, (or supervisor) more congruent with his/her own theoretical base and personal modus operandi." (p.237-238)

An example of this sabotage occurred in my supervision recently. In an agency where the narrative form of therapy is the recommended approach to treatment, an intern found that the focused questioning of this approach was not compatible with the need for open structure in a creative art therapy session. However, rather than throw the baby out with the bath water, she modified the narrative form and gave substance to the art therapy language. The combination proved effective, but it was necessary to be discreet with the agency supervisor in explaining the synthesis of the two ways of providing narrative.

## Personal and Anxiety-Provoking Issues

Often a neglected subject in the opening dialogue of supervision is the high anxiety aroused when the supervisor offers many alternate suggestions for proceeding with a case. No matter how considerately a supervisor uses language, it does feel like every move is criticized! The only preventative ploy I can suggest is to regularly check with trainees on how they feel about the support they are getting and whether or not they feel they "can't do anything right." Predicting this discomfort as a possible future problem often prevents the formation of the problem.

Personal issues are also a subject that must be reviewed from the beginning of the contract. Defining as completely as possible the parameters of supervision versus therapy is the responsibility of the supervisor. The limitations on supervision are recorded in detail in most ethical documents of mental health professions. Helping supervisees understand the concept of dual relationships and the supervisor's commitment to maintain the boundary between therapy and supervision, will not only educate the supervisee, but provide an additional sense of security for everyone.

Hines (1993) reflects on power and gender in defined roles:

> "....There seems to be agreement in the field regarding dual relationships where two or more socially defined roles are involved. This might be called an external dual role phenomena. I suggest another perspective concerning an internal role phenomena. Dual roles result from discrepancies in a supervisors internal perception of his or her role and the socially defined role of supervisor.... for example,he (a male supervisor) may give lip power to an egalitarian stance, but deny the power differential inherent at the beginning in senior supervisor and novice supervisee. (The denial places the supervisee in a paradoxical situation)... the internal dual role phenomena need as much attention as the external role." (p.3)

Goldenthal (1993) is concerned with maintaining a balance:

> "Many common ingredients (among varying theoretical orientations) involve achieving a delicate balance between competing pressures. Most supervisors agree that supervision needs balancing: (1) the needs of the supervisees and the clients: (2) supervisory responsibilities to supervisees and clients; (3) support for supervisees while challenging them, as appropriate; (4) a focus on the clients with a focus on the supervisee's personal growth; (5) discussions of immediate clinical and practical decisions regarding cases and more general clinical issues; and (6) the emphasis on technique and case management issues with discussion, directed readings, etc., designed to help supervisees develop their own coherent theoretical rational." (p.1)

## Dynamics Between Supervisor & Supervisee

A more difficult aspect to evaluate in supervision is on the personal level. Do each of you feel that your personalities will be compatible? The trainee may feel less empowered to reject the professional because he or she holds greater status. However, it is important that the question be raised: can we work together? Has our first meeting seemed to have answered your questions? Shall we confirm our mutual commitment to this process? It is not unlike the question I always ask my clients at the close of our first session.

It is unethical for any supervisor to continue supervision with someone to whom they feel a strong antipathy. No doubt this could be overcome with exploration of the transference, but supervisors are there for supervisees, not to work though their own issues. Much time can be wasted in a restricted emotional climate. It is wrong to accept money and trust from another colleague when you know that you are unable to give your best efforts because of some negative affect toward the other. Supervision is more than a commodity sold on the marketplace; it is the validation of the process of therapy and teaching.

An additional emotional component to the relationship is the matter of evaluation and/or grades. Pre-masters students in training will be concerned about their performance on two levels: one of growth, the other of survival in the program and their ego involvement in the grade. Post-graduate supervisees may not need or even desire an evaluation, however, regular feedback is important to the relationship. It is ethically irresponsible to continue with a supervisee who refuses to make changes that the supervisor feels are needed to benefit their clients. Short of radically unethical behavior, there is that gray area where sloppy work and lack of attention to detail becomes serious. If this behavior is not corrected after it has been brought to the trainee's attention, the relationship should be terminated. The supervisor should refuse to recommend the supervisee's performance or sign for his or her hours. This a radical stance, and would be perhaps a risky thing to do, but it should be considered and explored with counsel if there is any legal question involved. Again I repeat, the supervisor is responsible for his or her supervisee's therapeutic treatment of clients (Charney,1986).

I suspect that in no other relationship, except the therapist/client contract, does the experienced professional need to carefully examine their ethics, attitudes, prejudices and responsibilities toward another person. If supervision is the arena where the greatest learning can take place, conversely it is also the field where the greatest damage can be done. The supervisee is at risk because they are vulnerable in their discomfort as they begin to take on the mantle of directing clients on their quest for change. It is not easy to assume the position of therapist when one's recent identity has been student or trainee.

In some situations the supervisee is chronologically older than the supervisor. This reversal of role/authority must be addressed from the start of the relationship. Often both parties deny that it will be a problem; however, it may be a difficulty that is masked in many ways. One method of coping with this situation is to acknowledge that the younger is older in the field and the older can enjoy again the freedom of youth in the relationship. Good supervisors do not come in certain packages. All the variations of relationships will be found and common tensions are to be expected. Again, the burden of bringing the issue into the dialogue should come from the supervisor who can encourage or give permission to discuss *age*, which is often a taboo subject in a social setting.

## The Developmental Approach to Supervision

The notion of looking at the supervisory relationship through the lens of normal developmental cycles is appealing. This focus has been cogently described by Friedman and Kaslow (1989) in their article on developing the professional identity. They delineate six stages of development in this manner (paraphrased):

Stage one: Excitement and anticipatory anxiety. This stage is brief. It begins during the time the trainee becomes acquainted with the agency, and ends when she sees her first client.

Stage two: Dependency and identification. This stage begins as soon as the trainee is assigned a case. It ends when she realizes that she has a significant impact on a given client. Friedman and Kaslow describe the supervisee's emotional overload at this time, and their confusion, which restricts their willingness and abilities to reveal all their doubts concerning treatment.

Stage three: Activity and continued dependency. During this phase the authors believe that the intern moves from passivity and dependency to a more active, less dependent mode. The danger at this time is that the new therapist fluctuates between gross overestimation of her abilities, to an equally inaccurate underestimation of her skills. The supervisor's experience at this time is one of frustration and hope as he or she lives through a messy time of development.

Stage four: Exuberance and taking charge. The therapist now feels he or she is a therapist. The focus of supervision is on clinical matters and the trainee is secure enough to handle counter transference matters.

Stage five: Identity and independence. The trainee pulls away from the supervisor and often initiates a power struggle with the supervisor. This gradually moves toward a more measured evaluation of her/his strengths and those of the supervisor.

Stage six: Calm and collegiality. The calm arising from a secure sense of identity as a professional, an appreciation of her/his peers, senior staff, and supervisor. It also is a time to re-examine theoretical belief systems and reach out to other experiences. (p.29-45)

This brief recapitulation of Friedman and Kaslow's discussion of development does not do justice to the articulate essay they have written on this subject. The reader is urged to read the original for a complete appreciation of their hypotheses.

Others have described the development of supervisees. For example, Hess (1986) sees the development process of professional identity in these terms:

1). Inception—characterized by insecurity, dependency, and inadequacy; 2) Skill development—moving from dependency toward autonomy and adequacy; 3) Consolidation—the development of self confidence and the shift from conditional dependency to individuation; 4) Mutuality—a time of creativity and independent practice. (p. 51-68)

It is generally true that the earliest phase of supervision involves dependency, and rightly so. The learner must feel free to ask for help and acknowledge confusion and fear. It is how that dependency is gratified that is the moot question. A great strength that beginners bring to our profession is their refreshing vision, enthusiasm, and excitement when they first observe how the art product leads to therapeutic ends. It is that very child-like response to visual material that can be a real addition to the process of both the client's therapy and the supervisory relationship.

It is important for the supervisor to encourage and develop supervisees' skills in retaining their freshness while at the same time, combine it with concepts and techniques that will be available for future situations. The "visual knowing" of a child, the concrete view, the naive awareness of imagery, are strengths that many art therapists have joyfully preserved. Therefore, more experienced professionals must first see what they can learn from their students before intimidating them with the concepts and the visual knowledge that have been used in the past. Carl Whitaker (1989) believed that if the therapist is not learning and having some fun, then neither is the family in therapy. That certainly is true in supervision.

There is a limit however, to the child-like response. Success in using an art process has often resulted in a repetition of the same directive for subsequent therapeutic situations. The art does not 'work' unless it is tailored to the unique needs of that particular client or family. When repeating the same directive in another situation, the beginner can be disappointed in the failure of the intervention and label the client as resistant. In actuality, the trainee has inflicted an inappropriate suggestion on the participants in therapy. This same mistake can be repeated with media. For example, a miracle seems to have happened when the client was able to find the magazine collage picture that made concrete their internal distress in pictorial form. Yes, it was an important moment for the therapist with the client; however, the new supervisee may then over-use collage in other situations where this media will not effectively elicit the same reaction or could be counter productive. Media, like directives and language, must be particular to that moment in time for the therapy to work.

The attention to the setting and the context in which the art therapy is offered may be misunderstood by the beginner. Art tasks that may be effective in the outpatient clinic may be a disaster in the hospital. The variables are numerous. At times, a client may be more productive creating reflective art work at home and bringing it into the session. The art therapy intern may feel that he or she has not been *enough* of an art therapist if the client does not create something during the session. There is an issue of control in this situation and possibly an internal pressure to show the supervisor that he or she is able to inspire the client to be creative and to solve problems through art.

## Respecting the Art Product

A discussion of how client's art products are handled is important in the supervisory relationship. For example, if a molested child reveals abuse in the art product, this drawing should not go home until proper steps have been taken to protect the child and explore the molestation. The art expression may eventually be used as documentation of abuse against the perpetrator. Also, the youngster may be accused of tearing the family apart or lying about the abuse, feeling betrayed once again. There is no way of knowing the impact the art product will have on the family. The therapeutic alliance that provided comfort and protection for the molested child can be harmed beyond recovery by a supervisee who does not understand the consequences of keeping the child's drawings as confidential case records.

There are countless other circumstances in art therapy where an unpremeditated response or lack of confidentiality with the art product shows lack of respect. Displaying the client's art without serious consideration of the implications of turning a clinical product into a decorative display is anti-therapeutic. The novice may decide to display the art on an impulse, to show how the art conveys a message; however, it still can be destructive. Spontaneity differs from impulsivity; often the two modes of action are confused. To move on a clinical decision impulsively implies that one has put thoughtful judgment aside and acts without weighing the consequences. Spontaneity is defined as freedom from constraint or pressure, to act naturally, and is compatible with the therapeutic process. Both of these reactions may be valid under certain circumstances, but impulsive action does not fit the therapeutic ideal.

## Impact of Art Expressions on Supervisees & Supervisors

The undiluted impact of a traumatic image presented in art therapy is very difficult to handle at any stage of development, for the supervisor as well as the supervisee. For the neophyte it is an experience that may be painful, not only because of the client's anguish, but because the imagery may evoke, on a deeply personal level, parallel emotions or memories for the supervisee. The beginning practitioner should be allowed to process reactions and be actively supported. If the support invites over-dependency at a later stage, it is another matter—one that can be separated from the impact and emotional identification with the client's tragedy. This may be called "visual countertransference".

We must not forget that the reason that art therapy is such a successful therapy is because it has an evocative, informational power. How this stressful material is perceived by new practitioners is a sensitive matter and may be a stimulant to their own repressed difficulties. The supervisor should be aware that these times of fusion between the client's pain and the supervisee's pain is one that calls for delicate understanding and a time to resist entering into a therapy relationship with the trainee. The best insurance against forming a dual relationship is to be sure that supervisees have their own therapists who can handle these unusual situations. To become therapist and supervisor simultaneously is to defeat the purpose of therapy and supervision. The two roles must always be kept apart, even though the borders seem to touch.

## Time to Individuate

After some time has passed and sufficient clients have been seen, the progress of the supervisee often takes another turn. It is not unlike the bravado of adolescence. The symptoms come through in statements such as: "I already tried that approach", "That directive has been done before", "None of the clients are having any problems with me now" or "I really don't have anything to talk about today." Do these remarks sound familiar? This may not be the most rewarding period of supervision for the supervisor, but he or she can feel a sense of satisfaction that they have not encouraged a symbiotic dependency! This is the time to get into serious theoretical discussions. At an 'adolescent' phase the intellect is very lively. Here is the time to explore new concepts, to examine in what context a particular therapeutic move was successful and to challenge the established way of presenting therapy and push the supervisee to adventure in untried ground—to vary their approaches to therapy (Frantz, 1990 ).

The respect given by the supervisor to the trainee is important. Positive reinforcement is helpful, but caution must be observed. There is danger in the possibility that new courage may overlook old principles. The supervisor, at the time of the supervisee's adolescent behavior, must be attentive to his/her case reports and the recent developments with the client. In the excitement of newly earned freedom from their initial insecurities, the reporting of abuse, writing progress notes on time, and attending required meetings may be neglected by the intern. A few sessions in supervision should control the neglectful behavior.

Another aspect of individuation in the art therapy trainee is an inclination to move away from encouraging the use of art expression in the therapy. Just as the child revels in the pleasure of unstructured expression, adolescents become more self-conscious of their aptitude. Supervisees, in this adolescent phase, will wait until the absolutely *perfect* time arises for the absolutely *unique* directive to be offered. When that time comes, perfection is out of reach (as it always is), the session is over and the art has been forgotten. In essence, the trainee has used the intellectualization of adolescence to become a verbal therapist. Fortunately, growth continues and the basic drive for creativity both in their own lives and in the lives of the clients becomes again the dominant drive. Words and images will eventually find a balance in the art therapist's practice, especially with guidance from the supervisor at this time.

Sooner or later some aspect of feelings around authority figures will be the center of the dialogue and it seems most likely to occur in the adolescent phase. Defying the supervisor by taking counterproductive action with the clients, simply to demonstrate 'individuation' is unacceptable. An example of 'defiance' of a trainee was observed in this manner. When treating a family, the intern chose to see the child alone because she disliked the parents. Subsequently the mother began to feel replaced and resentful of the therapist and removed the child from therapy. The choice to see the child individually had been discussed and rejected in supervision. The consequences had been predicted. How the supervisee appraises his/her actions, or other incidents similar to this example, tells the supervisor in what stage of development the trainee remains.

The supervisor should encourage the move toward independent thinking and extinguish the need to act-out to achieve it. The first rule of supervision is: Any therapeutic action that results in a negative outcome for the client is unacceptable. Supervision is created for the benefit of the client's treatment and through that benefit the supervisee learns. The core of the supervisee's learning process is to understand this credo.

## Evaluating Client Art

How the supervisee acquires skills to evaluate the client's artwork also follows a pattern that can be seen through the same developmental lens described in the previous sections of this chapter. The supervisor encourages the supervisee to find the messages in the art, look for repetitive patterns, and evaluate the structure and the imagery. The beginner is given the opportunity to become immersed in the clients visual language. Then, the supervisor teaches how to refrain from imposing unsolicited observations upon the persons in treatment.

At the early stages of development there is a child-like glee in the discovery that the art really works but as in all 'growing up' the rules of restraint have to be learned. At later stages of development, the supervisee may wish to utilize a more structured art therapy directive, a projective test protocol or technical directives for achieving goals. This is a time when spontaneity takes second place. These formulated directives provide security, and in some cases are needed to succeed in treating specific populations; however, they have limitations. Limitations may consist of restricting the creative production of client art expressions, creating dependency on directives issued from the art therapist, or reinforcing the suspicion that the art is requested for diagnosis only. After this type of assessment process, the art therapy supervisor should question the use of a formula and explore with the trainee if it is used for the therapist rather than the client.

## The Challenge of Art in Therapy

There is an aspect of art therapy supervision that differs from other professions in mental health. While exploring client art work together with the trainee the supervisor must withhold the imposition of a final judgment about what is actually visually experienced in the art. This includes imagining you can see through the client's eyes. The biology of each human brain differs and because of that the visual receptors send singular visual images to each of us. We imagine that everyone else *sees* what we see, although that is not possible. In addition, one hemisphere of the brain has the ability to 'know' the world though silent visual images. The non-verbal message must remain silent until the verbal section of the brain gives words to the original visual impressions (Tinnin, 1991). Thus we engage both hemispheres of the brain for complete understanding.

These mysterious workings of our mind lend an aspect of uncertainty to any interpretation of the art. Therefore, the investigation of the client's art product in supervision must also take into account that there is a possibility that no two people see the image in exactly the same way. Each observer understands the art product based on a variety of interpretations.

It is important that supervisors and educators be receptive to these new concepts and push the exploration of the art into broader horizons. Tinnin (1991) said:

> "Creativity... is the fusion of the mental activity of the verbal and nonverbal brains. The magic in this process is the preservation of the nonverbal mental output in spite of the conscious illusion of unity and against the force of cerebral dominance...The nonverbal portion of the creative product is generally covert, but carries the effect of universality. It arises from the biologically given portion of the brain with its unsymbolized and uncensored primary process mentation. It reflects capacities for instantaneous, nonverbal thought that go far beyond the usual limits of the conscious mind" (p.353).

Supervisors sympathize with their supervisees' impatience to become competent. They must both accept that only with time do art therapists gain experience and the ability to tolerate the paradoxes of therapy and life. Supervisors cannot speed up progress for their trainees, but there are significant insights that can be reinforced. For example, in time it becomes apparent that the art work arises from the therapeutic process and that only in that context should therapists make suggestions for an art expression. Trainees will also come to know that clients who have been introduced to art making from the inception of treatment will not need to be coached to manufacture a drawing. The supervisee will understand that the imagery will flow from the conversation and that conversation will reflect the content of the art. Other times the art alone will be the dialogue, without words, and possibly responded to only by the next piece of art. Eventually, the enthusiasm of the early experience becomes fused with the restraint of the more experienced professional and the art therapist shares in the excitement of the clients' use of their personal creativity.

Lastly, trainees develop an appreciation that evaluation of the client is ongoing. What appeared to be true in the art of yesterday, may have evolved into a new view of reality that invalidates the previous truth. Evaluation and assessment as a component of treatment is a dynamic process. When it is used in a reductionist manner to give the therapist a sense of security, it assesses only her/his insecurities, not the client's.

## Maturation of the Supervisor

The final aspect of the developmental viewpoint has to do with the supervisor. Where is the supervisor on the continuum of growth? This is a question that each responsible supervisor should take into account and explore in their own therapy or with colleagues. Supervisors find themselves reflected in their trainees' work and if they have little sense of their own areas of struggle, they will be less able to help trainees find their own way. There is nothing wrong with knowing that you have retained a child, an adolescent, and a crabby parent within yourself—the wrong is in not controlling those parts of the self when they surface inappropriately. In fact, sharing the child can be essential in supervision. There is no substitute for laughter and pleasure in the relationship to make learning easier. Assuming the role of supervisor should become an opportunity to learn more about one's self in order to better co-create an optimum experience for both yourself and the trainee.

## Conclusion

The supervisory relationship is the nexus that binds the theoretical learning to the experiential practice of knowledge. The supervisor is the guide that encourages the new art therapist to move from neophyte to professional. Supervision exists in a unique world that is not therapy, but is therapeutic and educational. In this relationship both parties grow as they co-create opportunities for the supervisee's clients to receive treatment. Personal issues must be addressed before they interfere with this treatment. In spite of this closeness, the structure of supervision must not be weakened or confused by personal dynamics.

The complications of the supervisory relationship are countless, however, they can be controlled, explored, enjoyed and utilized as a positive learning experience. The goal of the supervisory experience is focused on the best possible therapy for the clients. When this is the aim of supervision there is clarity and positive, creative and pragmatic educational growth for the supervisee.

## References

Ard, B.N. (1973). Providing clinical supervision for marriage counselors. A model for supervisor or supervisee. *The Family Coordinators, 22*, 91-97.

California Association of Marriage and Family Therapists. (1990). *Practical applications in supervision: A manual for supervisors.* San Diego, CA: Author.

Charney, I.W. (1986). What do therapists worry about? A tool for experiential supervision. In F. Kaslow (ed.), *Supervision and Training.* (p.17-28). New York: Haworth Press.

Cohen,M., Gross,S.. & Turner,M. (1976). A note on a developmental model for training family therapists through group supervision. *Journal of Marriage and Family Counseling, 2,* 48-56.

Doehrman, M.J.G. (1976). Parallel process in supervision and psychotherapy. *Bulletin of Menninger Clinic., 40*(1),103-104.

Ekstein, R., & Wallerstein, R. (1972). *The teaching and learning of psychotherapy.* New York. Basic Books.

Frantz, T.G. (1990). Developmental stages in supervision: Implications for supervisors and administrators. *In CAMFT Manual for Supervisors.* (p.3-8-22). San Diego, CA: CAMFT.

Friedman,D. & Kaslow,J.N. (1986). The development of professional identity in psychotherapists: Six stages in the supervision process. In F.W.Kaslow (ed.), *Supervision and Training: Models, Dilemmas, and Challenges.* (p.29-50). New York: Haworth Press.

Gardner, M. H. (1980). Racial, ethnic and social class considerations in psychotherapy supervision. In, A.K.Hess (ed.), *Psychotherapy.* ( p.474-508). New York: Wiley & Sons.

Gillen, J.S. (1990). Different types of countertransference and the importance of addressing them in supervision. *In CAMFT Manual for Supervisors.* (p.3-156-160). San Diego, CA: CAMFT.

Goldenberg, I. & Goldenberg, H.(1991). *Family therapy; An overview.* Pacific Grove, CA: Brooks/Cole .

Goldenthal, P.(1994). A matter of balance, Challenging and supporting supervisees. *The Supervision Bulletin of American Association of Family Therapists.* Vol. VII. No. 2. p 1-2. Washington, DC.

Hess, A.K. (1980). *Psychotherapy supervision: Theory, research and practice.* New York: Wiley & Sons.

Hines, M. (1993).Dual aspects of a dual relationship. In *The Supervision Journal of American Association of Family Therapists.* Vol. VI, No. 1. p.2-3. Washington DC.

Kaslow, F.W. (1977). *Supervision, consultation and staff training in the helping professions.* San Francisco: Jossey-Bass.

Kaslow, F.W. (1986). *Supervision and training: Models, dilemmas, and challenges.* New York: Haworth Press.

Liddel, H., & Saba, G. (1982). Teaching family therapy at the introductory level: A model emphasizing a pattern which connects training and therapy. *Journal of Marital and Family Therapy, 8,* 63-72.

Nichols, W. (1988). Family therapy/education training: An integrative psychodynamic and systems approach. In. H.A.Liddle, D.C. Breulin, & R.C. Schwartz (eds.) *Handbook of family therapy training and supervision.* (p. 110-127). New York: Guilford.

Schwartz, R. (1987). The trainer-trainee relationship in family therapy training. In. H.A. Liddle, D.C. Breulin, & R.C. Schwartz (eds.) *Handbook of family therapy and supervision.* (p. 172-182). New York: Guilford Press.

Sluzki, C. (1979). Migration and family conflict. *Family Process*, 379-390.

Whitaker, C. (1989). *Midnight musing of a family therapist.* New York:W.W. Norton & Company.

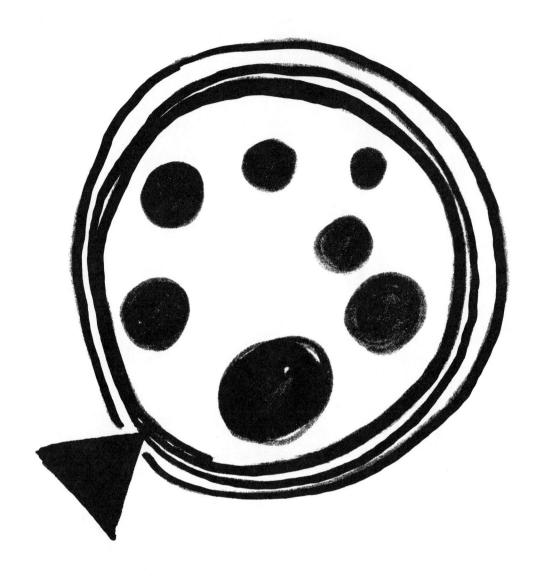

Can't get into the family.

# CHAPTER FOUR
## Supervision Case Study
by Shirley Riley

This chapter describes a year of supervision with a second year trainee enrolled in a marital and family therapy/clinical art therapy masters-level program. I teach several classes in this program and have been a faculty member for many years. In addition to the normal contractual arrangement I had with the trainee, she was aware that I was also being supervised as a supervisor. This was a requirement to attain the Approved Supervisor Certificate for the American Association of Marriage and Family Therapists. My supervision was conducted by my supervisor viewing videotapes made of supervisory sessions with this trainee and with others. The dual position of being a supervisor and simultaneously being supervised provided a unique quality to supervision; I learned more about supervision by experiencing a parallel position with the supervisee. I believe it proved advantageous to both of us.

Presenting this supervision case study is influenced by two considerations: 1) can teaching and supervision exist in an academic setting without being contaminated by a dual relationship? and 2) what can be learned by examining the trainee's innate strengths and weaknesses through a review of two of her client cases. These two issues offered both the supervisor and supervisee a new understanding and surprising outcomes. Looking carefully at this supervision allows me to explore the confluence of training, personality and guidance in a manner that is personally challenging.

## Providing Structure and Attempting to Forestall Difficulties

With this supervisee, as with all the students I have supervised, I first clarify my position as professor as separate from that of supervisor. I teach a first year class the semester before I assume the role of supervisor with a second year student. I acknowledge that I know the student in an academic relationship and have some acquaintance with her therapeutic skills based on her classroom performance and understanding of theory. During the first semester I am not committed to any particular person for future supervision. However, as a professor, I have become a "personality" in the eyes of the students, with all their projections, fantasies and anxieties about grading, as part of their *knowing* of me. On the positive side, the future supervisee also knows my current thinking in family theory, has seen me role-play and has been introduced to my preference for certain theoretical stances in the conduct of therapy—I come as no surprise.

When the trainee is assigned to me by the practicum coordinator, as the supervisor for his/her second year, two-semester practicum, many issues must be discussed. Generally speaking, the student is "honored" that I have been chosen for her or him, however, that honor has two edges: 1) the fear that I will not keep confidential from other faculty their 'shameful weaknesses' and that I will have unusual expectations for her or his performance; or 2) the trainee will exhibit a lack of trust because of some countertransference issues, often around persons in an authoritative role. Some students' desire working with me because of my experience and some are dismayed at what they perceive as an extra challenge. No matter what stance they take, I spend a good deal of time before the contract is culminated, attempting to bring all these issues to light. I am clear that if there is too much to overcome, we will not begin supervision. The discussion is rather like the guidelines for multicultural treatment. It is essential to confront differences and co-create a workable alliance. Still, there can be issues that will surface during the two semester relationship, having to do with anxiety that the supervision will be contaminated in some way by my position on the faculty. For myself, I find that I am more careful than usual in resisting the making of any personal inquiries and keeping a very clear boundary between supervision and friendship, and above all, therapy. Any dual relationship can be suspect.

Having addressed the basic structure of our relationship, the supervisee and I proceed with the physical arrangements of time, place, promptness, documentation, evaluations and 'permission to be a neophyte'. I also discuss the possibility that my help and dialogue will, in the beginning phase of learning, sound overcritical instead of supportive. It takes sensitive awareness on the supervisor's part to use language that is instructive and is cleansed of inferred negativity. Supervisors should look for unique strengths rather than weaknesses in the supervisees.

I also give the intern permission to fail if the failure is an issue recognized and puzzled over in supervision. Often the student's condemnation of him or herself is not one I agree with. It may just be that the clients' fluctuations of human behavior are patterns in the course of therapy to which the beginner is not accustomed. I often say the real failure is the lack of courage to examine a difficult issue, or the narcissistic stance of thinking one knows better than the client what is right for them. Putting the label of resistance on a client is an easy way to escape therapeutic responsibility!

During the course of supervision when it seems appropriate, I share some of my failures and client-difficulties with the trainee. I believe that supervision can be humanized and expanded if the supervisor can share their own clinical cases that shed light on the issues at hand. For that reason I believe that supervisors should be active in the field and experience work with clients in a parallel manner with the student in practicum. It is ideal if the supervisor is on staff at the trainee's practicum since both supervisor and trainee will be influenced by the larger system and the internal politics of the institution.

## A Supervisory Experience

The trainee, M., was my supervisee for a school year. She impressed me as a woman capable of thoughtful, intelligent exploration of theory and practice. She had a calm but affective persona with the strength to disagree and justify her own opinion in the classroom and she had a mature and graceful way of conducting herself. She had life experience and previous responsible jobs. M. was not married, nor did she have children. She related to her siblings and divorced parents, but seemed to have separated from her family of origin in an appropriate manner. She was in on-going personal therapy which I saw as a major plus. I felt that she would be an addition to the staff and further the status of art therapy treatment in the practicum to which she was assigned.

The clinical setting of the practicum was the family and child division of a county community mental health center. The family systems approach was recognized and there was a high regard for art psychotherapy. The family art therapist was given prime responsibility for family treatment, had full staff privileges and was not adjunctive. I had been senior staff there for seventeen years prior to my leaving the position to enlarge my scope of teaching and private practice. I am still retained as a supervisor/consultant, without pay. The familiarity with the setting provided comfort for both the trainee and myself.

Supervision was somewhat restricted with regard to video and audiotape equipment. A video camera was available at times and audio tapes were used with certain families, however, we relied primarily on the art therapy products which gave concrete witness to the sessions as well as progress notes, special documentation, and verbal reporting.

## Case Example One

This family was comprised of a single mother (age 42), recently separated (6 months) from her significant other, a relationship of one year. She had been divorced from her husband for three years. Her ex-husband had remarried, had a new baby and was living on the east coast. Living with the mother was a daughter (age 9), and a son (age 4). The problems reported by the mother were; 1) continuous tantrums by her son with no recognizable patterns, 2) feelings of extreme guilt because she believed she was a bad mother and 3) no longer having a father figure in the home. The recent separation from the boyfriend was motivated by the man's intolerance of the son, the daughter's childish behavior, and his desire to instigate severe punishment as discipline. To the mother's credit, she would not allow him to hurt the children.

In this family system the daughter acted as a surrogate mother to her brother and attempted to support her mother as an equal. The girl verbalized her anger at the mother for losing her father to another woman. She wanted to live with him and at the same time, wanted to stay with her brother. There was a great amount of conflict between mother and daughter because of this issue. The little boy seemed to be responding to all these changes and arguments with the emotional language of screams and tantrums. He could not be appeased when he began this behavior. The mother had attended many parenting classes, had a good education and a job, but her attitude toward the therapist was very challenging and abrasive. She was also extremely annoyed that she had an intern assigned to her case. Her personality and manner of presenting herself was the direct opposite of the supervisee.

## Role of the Therapist/Trainee

M. spoke in a quiet tone of voice. Her natural inflection raised her voice at the end of a sentence, as though she was asking a question. She had a difficult time sounding firm and making a statement rather than posing a question. M. looked younger than her years, but acted appropriately adult at all times. Her conceptual understanding of family theory was excellent, but the challenge of confrontations (no matter how restrained) with belligerent clients was an acknowledged problem. When the mother aggressively challenged her ability to help her son stop his tantrum behaviors, she was intimidated and felt defeated. Every suggestion M. offered was countered by a negative remark by Mrs. S. and M. felt that the mother knew more about parenting than she did. In fact, this probably was true. The mother said M.'s manner of speaking made her feel that the therapist was tentative and unsure and she threatened to leave therapy. My trainee was very discouraged and we spent a lot of time going beyond the aggressive, challenging behavior of the parent and into the realm of speculating why this attitude was so rigidly in place. One might speculate that M.'s delicate way of being a woman was the very thing the mother wanted for herself but also resented.

The clinical dilemma was in knowing how to reassure the mother that she was a good parent and still find a way to diminish the power the boy's temper tantrums held over the whole family. The mother felt that somehow her failure to stop the tantrums was tied in with the issue of losing men in her life. Her son spoke in baby talk, hung on to his sister inappropriately and had tantrums three or four times a day. M. made an effort to identify with the mother, but was rejected. We attempted to offer parenting skills around the tantrum behavior, but Mrs. S. had "read every book and had attempted every intervention".

Although the three were willing to draw together and accomplish art tasks, the products were superficial and only the daughter was invested in the art therapy experience. We had hoped to address the missing father through the art expressions but that did not happen until later in the therapy. Finally, after several months of the family's spotty attendance, we decided that the three members of the family had established a rigid pattern and that it would take a strategic approach to help them solve the problem. I discussed with the trainee a variety of reasons that the mother might hold such guilt and why she was becoming progressively more incompetent. We recognized that with tantrums it is nearly impossible to discover the original reason for the anger. The behavior now had a life of its own and had become a powerful tool for control. Evidently this anger/control syndrome, in another form, had existed in the trainee therapist's family of origin and thus made it even harder for her to intervene in a helpful manner.

Together we devised a strategic plan to offer to the mother. We acknowledged that the boy had very strong feelings about something. At four years old, he did not have the words to express this complicated feeling and therefore used the language of tantrums. We respected this need to express his emotions. The mother was reassured that she had been supportive and not repressed his need to emote. This anxiety was a constant fear that restrained her from stopping his behavior. We limited our strategic suggestion to a change in the location of the tantrums. This was rationalized as 'so he could be safe'. He was to be helped into a room in the house that was danger free and encouraged to continue his tantrum. The door was to be closed and the mother would sit outside the door until he was through. She felt she could not physically move any further away because of her guilt, so we prescribed the ongoing interactions and behaviors. The mother's closeness also gave the boy the reassurance that she was supportive. When he was quiet she opened the door, held him and consoled him, promising him that some day words would come. In the meantime the mother would be patient. The older sister was not to intervene or help her brother.

This ritual seemed to take care of the Mrs. S.'s anxiety about failings as a mother and gave the boy 'permission' to throw the tantrum, thus taking away the control issue. Gradually the behavior ceased except on rare occasions. The hardest part of this intervention was to coach the supervisee to speak in a firm, even manner inspiring confidence and controlling the 'question' inflection in her voice. It was interesting to me that this intelligent supervisee understood the complicated relationships but needed to learn how to mold her behavior to fit the expectations of the family. Stepping outside to observe ourselves is very difficult. I needed help in this situation also. I had become accustomed to my supervisee, liked her and felt that we had a profitable time discussing cases. I did not hear the question in her voice any longer. It was my supervisor who stopped the video tape and ran it over several times, challenging me to pick up this subtle inflection in her verbal delivery. I was grateful for his observation.

I believe that it is a delicate situation to help a trainee with personal mannerisms without crossing over into a personal association or invading therapeutic territory that is inappropriate in the supervisory relationship. In this case, there was a willingness on her part to see how an incorrect message was being received by this mother, based on her erroneous assumptions about the vocal tonality. Recognizing this, which had little to do with her therapeutic skills, gave the supervisee an observant look at the situation. My lack of awareness was also discussed and that added to the desire for change. When the therapist/trainee modified her delivery and assumed a more authoritative tone, the mother heard the assurance that she needed. The therapeutic connection to the family improved and this reinforced the supervisee's gratification at making the change.

## Case Example Two

The second family consisted of a Latina mother and her two daughters. The father had been killed in a gang shooting a year before. Since that time the older daughter (age 13) 'had done nothing right', according to her mother. The mother berated and criticized her constantly. She kept up a nonstop dialogue of angry complaints and although some of them were realistic, most were normal adolescent behaviors that she misinterpreted. The younger girl (age 10) had gone to live with an aunt most of the week and had disengaged from this conflict as much as possible. Although this daughter had escaped direct attack from the mother, she still was reflecting the conflicts in the home by her failing school performance and a generally depressed affect. The depression served her well because in this family depression was considered good behavior—it was quiet and withdrawn. The mother had recently been hospitalized twice for suicidal threats. She refused medication and was deeply depressed and agitated. Meanwhile, the older daughter had become desperate, left school because she was a problem to the teachers and had run away from home. As with many Hispanic families with large extended family relationships, she had run from one relative's home to another. Recently the father's best friend who was close to the family had also been killed in a drive-by shooting. The death revived the fear and grief over the father's death which was ever present in the family's conversation but had no resolution. This family was torn apart by internal and external trauma.

## Role of the Therapist/Trainee

This case posed many pathological problems and was handled in a superior way by M. The suicidal threats of the mother and the progressive decompensation of the mother's controls and logical thinking capacities were a real threat to herself and her children. The beginning family contact was one of very irregular attendance and the supervisee swung from self-blame to client-blame. This was the time to educate the supervisee about the realities of a poverty and grief-stricken widow, who, in her culture, never had leadership responsibilities for her family. The murder of her husband left her devastated in many ways. The situation had to be seen in the cultural environment in which it existed. The mother had lost her security, her dependent position, her status as woman (married vs. widow) and was forced into a 'daughter' role with her parents. With her fragile inner strength she found relief by projecting her fears and angers onto her daughter, the closest witness to her tragedy. In the belief system of her family she was not expected to assume a male authoritarian role and yet, the school and social services demanded just the opposite. This taxed her frail resources beyond their capacity to function.

My supervisee was able to fully entertain these complicated family interactions. She spent many hours integrating a non-judgmental method of approaching this tense situation. I helped the trainee to understand that this mother should not be 'liberated' to the degree that she became an outsider to her own culture. The trainee supported the client when it was necessary to seek emergency hospitalization. When the client felt at risk and threatened suicide, M. sought additional supervision with clinic staff to insure protection for both the mother and her daughter. When M. realized that the mother had very little psychological support from her family she devised, on her own, a network home visit. Her goal was to enlist the extended family in the treatment and gain further understanding. The family welcomed this personal interest and nine members assembled. The entire family drew pledges to the older daughter and her mother that offered specific support and approval. They pledged their help because of the therapist's gracious manner and official position. They took seriously the mother's mental distress. The family was very taken by the supervisee's manner of speaking that inferred a question, which they considered to be respectful and in deference to their judgment.

At this meeting, the family helped the mother choose to attend the day treatment programs at the clinic. The daughter was kept within the family boundaries and no longer had to bear the brunt of her mother's distraught projections. My supervisee could then terminate (her practicum was ending) with the satisfaction that the family was being attended to in the best manner available in our community. In this very brief review of a complicated case, theory, case management and cross-cultural understanding were all involved. The very traits of the trainee that were less successful with the first family were a strength in making a strong therapeutic connection with the second.

## Conclusion

I learned from this supervisory relationship and I learned from my position of being observed by another supervisor. I do not believe that I have ever so clearly addressed the fact that each of us have many ways of presenting ourselves to the world. I examined my own treatment style and realized how I use certain modes of relating with each clinical situation. I listened to my own verbal delivery and how it might impact the therapy. These thoughts added one more dimension to the teaching, learning and supervising relationship, and enlarged my scope of understanding the complications of treatment and supervision.

I appreciated that seeking consultation and supervision is never inappropriate, even after years of experience and especially if the supervisor you choose is talented, as mine was. He was able to see me in a way I could not see myself. As I shared his observations with my trainee we both could take advantage of the parallel process in supervision. I reconfirmed that the gift of being supervised should not be restricted only to the beginner. The advanced therapist may be renewed and recommitted to the process of therapy when his/her work is attended to by a colleague.

_These case examples are a combination of experiences. The names and circumstances have been altered to protect confidentiality of both the trainees and the clients. I am indebted to Dr. Clarence Hibbs for his supervision and guidance through the AAMFT Approved Supervisor process._

_S.R._

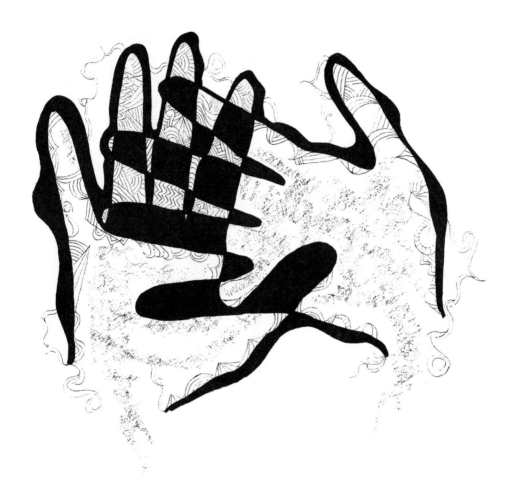

Supervision... is a chance to gain knowledge from my own experience... a place to learn about my place in the practice of art therapy. Supervision is not always comfortable and pleasant. I feel challenged to push myself, assert myself, and sometimes prove myself...

# CHAPTER FIVE

## Supervising Difficult Supervisees
by Cathy A. Malchiodi

This chapter explores some of the problems that supervisors may face in their supervisory work with trainees. As someone who has been supervising for quite a few years, I have not only had my share of memorable success stories, but also my share of mistakes and misgivings. I have chosen to focus more closely on the problematic aspects of supervision because these are often the experiences where the greatest opportunities for learning present themselves. Readers may recognize with private chagrin many of these dilemmas in working with difficult students from their own history as supervisors. A good deal of my real learning to supervise, advise, mentor and teach has come from revisiting my own fumblings and I imagine that many other professionals would agree that their errors have also been some of their greatest teachers.

As a preface to this section, it is important to realize that many of the problems that one has in supervising others are often a result of initially not having good training in supervision, particularly in the area of supervising problematic or difficult students. In my case, much of the earliest supervision I received was fairly unsophisticated and often uninformed. My supervisors simply were never trained to supervise, did the best they could given the circumstances, and did not think to forewarn me of any of the many possibilities for error and misjudgment in the supervisory relationship.

Also, as with many of my peers, it did not even dawn on me that effective supervision was a skill that required training and specific knowledge until I was well into practicing as a professional and was faced with supervising trainees on the job or as part of an academic training program. Needless to say, the variety of dilemmas that could occur within the framework of supervision was not immediately apparent to me because of this lack of training and mentoring. Additionally, of the articles available on the generalities of supervision with trainees in my field and related disciplines, very few presented any helpful or practical discussions about dealing with problematic aspects of supervision or problematic students. Therefore, the following discussion attempts to look at some of the situations in supervision that are perplexing, difficult, and often confounding, and can raise questions about a trainee's ability to practice as a therapist and effectively work with clients.

## Problematic Dynamics in Supervision

It is obvious that one of the most important components of supervision is the interpersonal dynamic between the supervisor and supervisee. Part of this dynamic is a direct result of the use of evaluation and feedback by one person (the supervisor) with another (the student/supervisee) for the purpose of teaching, skill improvement, communication of expertise, enhancement of the therapist/trainee's identity, etc. The other part of the dynamic evolves from how the trainee responds to the supervisor and the learning experience offered through supervision. This component of the relationship can present some very real problems to be solved and questions to be answered by the supervisor, particularly if the student is difficult, ill-equipped to undertake clinical work or has personal problems that affect client contact. Since the former dynamic is the subject of many of the chapters in this book, this discussion focuses on the latter, the problematic trainee and how this affects the supervisory relationship.

Reactions of trainees to supervision have been observed by many authors (Carrigan, 1994; Edwards, 1993; Wilson, 1981; Wilson, Riley, & Wadeson, 1984). One simple list of behaviors that impressed and informed my understanding of the supervisee is noted by Kadushin (quoted in Edwards, 1993) who described several ways that students may try to handle supervision. He noted the following three strategies:

1. Flattering the supervisor (e.g. be nice to me because I am nice to you).

2. Attempting to redefine the supervisory relationship as a social relationship (e.g. evaluation is not for friends).

3. Extreme self-criticism aimed at eliciting sympathy and minimizing the opportunity for the supervisee's work to be critically examined by others, including the supervisor (e.g. heading them off at the pass). (p. 66)

I think everyone who has supervised experiences the first dynamic—flattery. After all, everyone wants to be liked by others, particularly by those who are their mentors such as supervisors or teachers. Excessive praise and adulation's are typical, and on occasion even little gifts and gestures. Supervisors themselves may also play the flattery game with trainees, particularly if they are concerned about getting a good evaluation for their record or promotion. For example, many supervisors, in their confusion, naivete, or fear, simply avoid the task of giving criticism or negative feedback, finding it is easier to be 'liked' or they are simply lazy about addressing or confronting problems that are apparent in trainees. Supervisors and supervisees in graduate training seminars are particularly vulnerable to this dynamic because the former will be eventually evaluated by the trainees and the latter will eventually be graded by the supervisor.

The second response identified by Kadushin is a little more complex, (attempting to redefine the supervisory relationship as a social relationship), but is also commonplace. Many supervisors grapple with social boundaries and role definitions, particularly if students are older or of similar age, and who are therefore adult learners rather than traditional students. A few years ago I supervised a graduate student who described herself as an adult, lifelong learner. When she came into the training program she was close to 50 years old and many years older than me. The age discrepancy is common in training and is an aspect that may or may not have effected the dynamic between teacher and student. However, in this case, what was more troublesome than her age was her style of 'being' a student. She did not see herself as a learner per se, but someone who was already advanced in her understanding and therefore, was intellectually equal to her instructors—at least in her mind. In order to reinforce this sense of equality, she usually subtly began to establish a social dynamic with the instructor; first, by finding opportunity to be with teacher during coffee breaks during class; then later asking for lunch appointments to discuss a paper or project; and finally, making phone calls to the instructor's home for advice. She was quite adept at creating a series of social interchanges that confused the teacher/student boundaries necessary to keep objectivity in the relationship.

Unfortunately, I was unwittingly lured into the dynamic that she desired. When I attempted to re-establish appropriate boundaries, all-out rebellion began involving her accusing me of not being available outside of class, despite my availability for appointments during the greater part of three days each week in my office. However, a more professional relationship was uncomfortable for her; what she needed was for me to be available in settings where she could feel that we were buddies rather than student and teacher.

The easiest way to address this type dynamic is to prevent its occurrence to begin with—as I wished I had. Establishment of boundaries is obviously key to preventing this situation in the first place: time limits for scheduled meetings, no calls at home unless an emergency, and keeping interactions professional through a written contract. I have heard many a supervisor and educator eventually come to the conclusion that these types of limitations are essential, not only for the student's sake, but also to prevent the supervisor being taken advantage of and to allow one a personal life outside of school or clinic.

In addition to a social relationship, a student may try to redefine the role of supervisor into one of personal therapist. As discussed in other parts of this text, this is a dynamic that is often difficult to avoid and many think that it is ultimately impossible to completely circumvent. Often trainees may unknowingly bring unresolved personal problems into therapy, thus luring the supervisor into providing a little counseling to soothe their woes. Despite the troublesome aspects of blurred boundaries and roles, there are other repercussions of allowing this permutation of the supervisory relationship to go too far. For example, when a supervisor acts like a counselor and then reverts to acting like an instructor rather than counselor, things can get uncomfortable. The student may then balk at any attempt of the supervisor to be a teacher and trainer, such as in the evaluative areas of the relationship (assessing the trainee's progress) and may feel hurt if anything less than positive feedback is given (e.g. now you have to give me a A or a positive evaluation).

With reference to the third area that Kadushin mentions (e.g. self-criticism), I have had more supervisees who actually have the opposite problem: they have an irrational fear of criticism of any kind. These trainees are often mortally wounded by the slightest hint of negative feedback, or are stunned when they are told that there is always room for improvement in one's clinical skills. One dynamic in art therapy that may contribute to this is the belief that all art of any kind or quality is acceptable. Encouraged by this traditional paradigm of the field, students may also wish hopefully that all types of writing, research, and clinical work will be acceptable and are upset when that is not the case.

Here is a more specific example: A trainee entered a graduate program with what was judged to be a strong aptitude for visual art and a long record of acceptance of her artwork in various exhibitions. As an undergraduate she was able to achieve an excellent academic record, however, becoming a therapist and integrating materials from counseling and psychology was not something that came easily to her. She also displayed a personality unsuited to therapeutic interaction: rather reserved and unapproachable, something that is acceptable in the personality of an artist, but not conducive to being a therapist and displaying empathy to others. A supervisor can try to help a trainee overcome personality problems, but if these characteristics are common to the student's approach to people in general, they may be impossible to change (Wilson, 1981).

The student's irrational fear of criticism eventually became so great that she struck out at anyone that even hinted of criticizing her—supervisors, teachers and even other students. In reality she knew that she was ill-equipped to do therapeutic work with clients, in fact did not even enjoy it, but was insistent that she had the same level of skill as a therapist as she did as a successful artist. Mollon (1989) notes that:

> "Trainees inevitably suffer injuries to their self-esteem and self-image when finding that they are floundering; the capacity to withstand these narcissistic blows, perhaps with the aid of supervision, is a crucial factor in whether or not the trainee can learn to practice effective psychotherapy." (p. 113)

In this case, the trainee eventually graduated from the program, going on to doing some work with clients briefly, then going back to her original talent for creating her own art. I think that in many cases where trainees are truly unsuited to being therapists (and truly unhappy), they often end up leaving the profession before too long. The unfortunate situation is that they have invested a great deal of time and money in their training and education, only to find out that it was not really what they wanted to or were skilled in doing. In the case of this trainee, she was academically proficient and exhibited no serious problems in her work with clients; she expected, as many who come to art therapy from an art background, that this would be a satisfactory career change, offering her an opportunity to remain in touch with the arts as well as be financially rewarding. The only missing component was the more subjective quality of being a naturally empathetic and helping individual. It is this type of quality that is often difficult to assess during initial training and hard to explain to a trainee who is lacking in it. Hopefully, supervisors and/ or advisors facing the situation described above will be able to sensitively explain to a trainee early on that he or she may not be a candidate for nor happy in a career as a therapist.

## Other Issues that Affect the Supervisory Relationship

Another issue that seems common to the dynamics between supervisors and supervisees is the aspect of denial that trainees are experiencing any difficulties in their clinical work or learning. For example, art therapy students because their learning has often come from the arts and humanities and not so much from the hard sciences, may have problems in clinical areas of understanding, as well as in technical writing and research. One trainee very quietly denied for most of a semester that he was not making a passing grade in a required class that covered personal appraisal and diagnostic categories, despite my weekly inquiries in the supervisory seminar. Other students who were also taking the course complained vociferously about the difficulty of the course (and the instructor!), seeking help in supervision in understanding the material. In retrospect, I suppose that student's cultural background and competition with another very bright female student who was also taking the class, and getting an A, created this denial. This passive behavior on the part of the trainee placed the unfortunate onus on the supervisor to investigate the situation. Since his progress in the course was confidential, I was not informed that he was failing until I received a notice from his professor who thought I should know his status since the course was required for graduation. This set up an even more uncomfortable task in supervision of confronting the denial. As a supervisor it also had me wondering what else the student might not be telling me, placing me in a very awkward position.

This brings up another distressing issue that supervisors must often face: whether or not they can write a recommendation—for the purpose of credentials or a job—for a trainee in their charge. Students often perceive supervisors and instructors, as owing them a recommendation at the termination of training, perhaps a recommendation for professional status in the AATA or other professional association, for entrance into another training program, or for employment. Many students who have problems academically, clinically, or both, still go on to graduate because of university policy on probationary periods. As a supervisor you may be aware of serious problems that do not necessarily show up through grades or other reports, but are nonetheless worrisome. For example, could a supervisor comfortably give a written recommendation to a student who displays personality traits that in the future could jeopardize a client's welfare? A case in point that comes to mind involved a student who plagiarized a large portion of a final research project. The supervisor and thesis committee chair to the project had to confront the student on the issue of plagiarism and see that the situation was rectified. However, even after such an incident is rectified, can one feel comfortable writing a positive evaluation of this supervisee? This and other situations can be quite difficult for supervisors to determine, especially if a student's behavior has caused the supervisor to have grave doubts about a trainee's personal ethics or judgment.

## Causes to Terminate Placement and Supervision

What about the really serious problems that students display during training? Wilson (1981) noted the following behaviors that would justify possible termination of an internship, practicum and supervision:

1. physical injury to a client, a fellow student, or anyone else at the placement;

2. inappropriate behavior in a placement that is disruptive to the functioning of the agency and/or to its clients (e.g. a trainee losing emotional control; sexually seducing a client; intoxication or drug abuse);

3. psychotic behavior that disturbs others or is a danger to the trainee or others (e.g. psychotic break, overt hostility, paranoia, severe depression or active hallucinations and delusions);

4. illegal or immoral behavior (e.g. trainee caught stealing agency supplies or altering clients records). (p. 100 )

Although these incidents are rare, they do occur and supervisors must be clear in their handling of such occurrences since client welfare is often at stake. For example, I once decided to terminate supervision when I discovered that a trainee had forged a letter of recommendation from another staff member as part of his application to a graduate training program. Although the incident was later resolved, my feeling was that I could no longer trust this individual to tell me the truth under any circumstances. This problem left me wondering if what he reported to me about his clinical work was true. I also did not want to take the risk of personal liability as his supervisor should he do something similar, and illegal, again.

A fellow supervisor reported to me that a trainee in his charge had a breakdown during training that caused her to be hospitalized in a psychiatric unit for over a month. The breakdown was caused by unresolved issues of childhood abuse and addictive behaviors. This is not a common occurrence, but one I hear my peer colleagues discuss frequently since it creates a dilemma in how to proceed with the trainee's academic program. In some cases, students are admitted who have unresolved issues of past abuse or may have had severe, life-interfering experiences with depression, eating disorders, or drug addiction. Although their interests in becoming a therapist often stem from experiences in therapy, these unresolved issues and conditions may become unmanageable and may threaten their work with clients. The supervisor is put in the uncomfortable bind of both protecting client welfare, the prime directive, and dealing with some pretty overwhelming problems in the supervisee.

On the other hand, training and supervising students with past or even recurring emotional problems does bring up some core issues about how we as professionals see therapy in general. Do we believe that therapy works?

Do we believe that people who receive intervention for emotional problems can and do recover, and go on to lead productive lives? And do we see supervisees who have experienced emotional problems as able to undertake or return to school or a practicum? The answers to these questions are difficult, but ones that supervisors are forced to face. It is difficult to give unbiased responses to these questions—often as difficult as it is to resist becoming the troubled supervisee's counselor or confidant.

In the case of the aforementioned individual, she had not divulged a history of past abuse to her supervisor and other problems in her life that still remained largely unresolved. These problems posed a threat to her clinical work. Because of her problems, it was obvious to several supervisors that she was not effective in her work with clients. However, by university policy she could not be dismissed from the training program because academically she had passed a probationary period. In this case, dismissal could also be treated as discriminatory. A patent solution to trainees with emotional problems often is to require that they go into therapy for help. However, within most training programs it is not permissible to ask a student to go to therapy, not only because it is impossible to order someone into therapy, but also because it compromises the choice, privacy and confidentiality of therapy.

Fortunately, in this case, the supervisor was able to eventually terminate the supervisory relationship with her, based on her continued use of inappropriate interventions with clients which were verified by other clinicians on-site. It was unpleasant and confrontational, but the supervisor felt far too uncomfortable, given the possibilities for client harm and his own liability, to continue in his capacity which involved ultimate responsibility for those with whom the trainee worked. In cases such as the one I have described, my only suggestion is to keep accurate records of the trainee's work and if possible, supervise with a team where other professionals can verify your observations of the trainee's inadequacies. If an academic program is involved, the supervisor and the school must be in constant communication from the beginning of the placement and particularly if problems arise.

Even if problems are addressed appropriately, there still may be repercussions for the supervisor who confronts a trainee with either minor or serious problems in performance. Rumors and distortions may circulate among other students. They may wonder if they are next in line for criticism, seeing an instructor or supervisor confront or even dismiss a trainee. The supervisor may feel anxious about actions taken and negative feedback from trainees—this fear alone has stopped many supervisors from making critical responses to students. The supervisor may even question his or her decisions. Again, it is always helpful to get consultation and a reality check from professional peers when uncomfortable situations with trainees arise.

Lastly, there are several questions that when answered may be helpful in understanding supervisor-supervisee dynamics and possible pending problems. These may be helpful in understanding your own reactions and observations: 1) Would you be willing to hire this trainee? 2) If you were a client, would you want to be served by this trainee? In several of the cases mentioned (e.g. the student without the aptitude for becoming a therapist or the trainee with serious emotional problems) there is reason to believe that the student's clinical abilities may not be sufficient, or even prove harmful to clients. 3) Or, to look at it in another way, is the student's behavior particular to the situation, or is it something that will repeat itself in other circumstances? In the case of the student who was deceptive about his failing grade and the trainee who plagiarized material, the answer may be difficult to determine. However, these incidents may create enough doubt in a supervisor's mind to question whether or not a trainee is reliable, forthright and honest in his or her actions and intentions.

## Addressing Serious Problems in Supervision: Some Practical Guidelines

Many of the problems described in this chapter can be avoided through clearly defined guidelines for performance, skill acquisition, and competencies at the beginning of the supervisory relationship. When a supervisor is required to give a grade to a trainee for his or her clinical work, the supervisor is also serving in the capacity of an instructor and should clearly state on paper or in a syllabus:

1) How evaluation will take place; for example, in the case of a graduate trainee, attendance and participation in a weekly supervisory seminar, weekly presentation of one set of client progress notes, one case presentation to the class following a designated format, successful completion of a specified amount of practicum/internship hours.

2.) When or at what intervals will evaluation occur; for example, a written progress evaluation will be given to the student at the midpoint in the supervisory seminar, a final grade and summary of progress will be given at the end of the internship.

3) On what objectives the evaluation will be based; for example, a written set of objectives may include any or all of the following: ability to present case materials according to guidelines, ability to develop treatment plans, effective charting/progress notes, understanding of ethical principles and legal ramifications guiding clinical practice and appropriate use of supervision.

Within an academic setting, supervisors who feel a student is at risk of

91

failing are generally required to file some sort of a notification form that is given to the student, the coordinator of field placement, faculty advisor, and/or program director. This is often followed up by having a meeting with the student, supervisor and anyone else pertinent to the student's academic and clinical work.

Supervisors who work outside a school or training program (such as those who work with postgraduate interns) may have a more difficult time with problematic students since they are often outside an established network of other professionals. For this reason, evaluation of a trainee may be a little more difficult. In some cases, the agency at which the trainee is working may have developed guidelines for evaluation, but more than likely the supervisor is responsible for setting the structure and method of feedback and the objectives for the trainee's successful participation. Again, it is important to get as much of this down on paper, either in the form of requirements for the trainee (e.g. meeting times, paperwork expected, assignments) or a written contract containing both supervisor and supervisee expectations. The establishment of definable goals, objectives and expectations early in the relationship will prevent or solve many difficulties that arise later on in the experience.

Lastly, despite the supervisor's best efforts and intentions, there unfortunately will be times that a student's clinical work has serious flaws, a personality that is unsuited to success as a therapist, or at worst, actions which are unethical or illegal. All of these outcomes are of great concern to a supervisor, since a supervisor is responsible not only for the trainee, but also the clients that the trainee serves. Given this circumstance, the supervisor should immediately get feedback and consultation from other peer professionals, especially those who are familiar with the student's work and may be able to help the supervisor plan a course of action to address his or her concerns.

## Final Thoughts

Carrigan (1993) observed that "supervision is an unequal relationship in which interns have little freedom to make choices." Supervisors do have a great deal of perceived power and are capable of both appropriate and inappropriate use of this power. However, they also bear the brunt of the responsibility in the dynamic between supervisor and trainee. They are not only accountable for the training and mentoring of clinical skills in their supervisees, they are also responsible for the welfare of their supervisees' clients. This is a serious circumstance and one that must be not be taken lightly. Unfortunately, at one time or another in the life of a supervisor a trainee will come along who has some serious difficulties, is less than stellar as a clinician, or perhaps does something considered illegal or harmful to clients. With regard to the latter, a specific chapter has been included in this book concerning the liability of supervisors for their supervisees (see Chapter 14).

I also want to point out that Carrigan's observation does not account for the instances when a supervisor has an irresponsible, misguided, or even manipulative student. She also does not account for the volatile student that may sue the supervisor for frivolous reasons. Just as clients may have strong reactions to therapists, supervisees may have similar reactions to supervisors. As mentioned throughout this chapter, there are a great many variables involved in the supervisory relationship and supervisees may see the relationship far differently than the supervisor. There is unfortunately always a possibility that a supervisee may not meet the standards of training and the supervisor should be well aware of the ramifications of confronting, working with, or living with unacceptable trainee performance. Because of rules within a training program or institution, problematic trainees may not be easily dismissed or placed in internships elsewhere. Thus, it is not always possible to say in all circumstances that a supervisor has the upper hand or ultimate authority and can easily become a victim in the balance of power as can any supervisee.

In closing this chapter that focuses largely on the troublesome aspects of the supervisory relationship, it is important to remember that supervision can provide some of the most gratifying experiences in one's professional life as a therapist. Anyone who has ever supervised for any length of time has had to deal with unsatisfactory performance, questionable behaviors in supervisees, and a great many ethical dilemmas. However, in contrast, there is a certain gratification that comes over time when one learns to deal with many of these problems effectively. Part of this satisfaction comes from the knowledge that one acquires over the years in working with students and trainees; another part comes from seeing their progress in clinical work, watching the development of a professional identity, landing a job or promotion, giving a successful inservice or conference presentation, designing research, or receiving their calls to ask a question or get an opinion as a peer professional. Those are the rewards that minimize the problems and dilemmas, bringing the realization that one's efforts as a supervisor have paid off.

## References

Carrigan, J. (1993). Ethical considerations in a supervisory relationship. Art Therapy: *Journal of the American Art Therapy Association, 10,* 130-135.

Edwards, D. (1993). Learning about feelings: The role of supervision in art therapy training. *The Arts in Psychotherapy, 20,* 213-222.

Wilson, L., Riley, S., & Wadeson, H. (1984). Art therapy supervision. Art Therapy: *Journal of the American Art Therapy Association, 1* (3), 100-105.

Wilson, S. (1981). *Field instruction: Techniques for supervisors.* London: Macmillan.

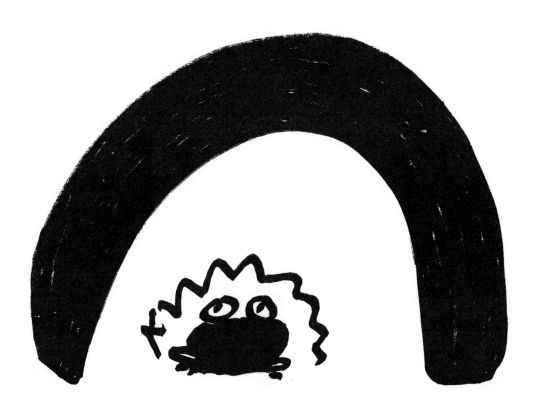

Overwhelmed in the session by the client's depression.

# CHAPTER SIX

## Integrating the Art Process into Supervision
by Cathy A. Malchiodi

This chapter offers some suggestions for using experiential work in supervisory sessions or as 'homework' between meetings with a supervisor. As noted in Chapter One the development of experiential ways of learning came from the area of interpersonal process work, a philosophy which emerged from the work of Rogers (1957) and other humanistic therapists. Although many art therapy educators and supervisors may think that they invented the idea of experiential learning, it really has its roots in humanistic approaches to both therapy and teaching.

For art therapists and art therapy educators, it seems natural to include art making within supervision and training. It is a way for trainees to explore theoretical material, clients, clinical issues and personal perspectives. It is also a way to help trainees stay in touch with the art process to some extent and to infuse the experience of art making into the framework of clinical training.

Art making is a potent modality through which one can sort out reactions to new situations, new identities (e.g. becoming a therapist), new clients or new ways of thinking. These complex feelings about clinical work are often difficult to verbally articulate early in training, especially when students are just starting to learn about transferential reactions, professional roles, the dimensions of client behaviors and working within clinical, community or other practicum settings. Art making may also be used to problem-solve; often art experiences help a trainee to visually explore particularly complex issues that involve the interaction of the therapist-trainee and the client or agency. For example, when a trainee reacts strongly to a client (either overwhelmingly positively or negatively), examining that dynamic through art may add some additional unknown or unarticulated information that was not previously communicated in the supervisory session.

## Some Considerations for Using Art Making Within Supervision

Possibly the most important reason for using art making within supervision is to allow the art therapist-in-training to connect didactic learning with the process of art making. This experience not only reinforces the importance of art as a way to learn about art therapy and understand clients, but also as a way of self-exploration for the therapist. It may also reinforce and strengthen the personal identity of an art therapist/trainee who is insecure in a practicum or internship where other professionals may not fully understand the use of art in clinical, medical or social services settings.

However, despite the usefulness of art making in training, it is important to consider some parameters of using art making with supervisees. Many of the same instincts that therapists have about using art with clients also apply to assigning art experiences to supervisees. Sensitivity to the supervisee's stage of development and current struggles with clients and self are extremely important considerations. In using art making to illuminate learning and stimulate thinking, supervisors must also think carefully about the impact of these types of assignments in terms of appropriateness, timeliness and needs of the trainee. In reality, supervisors must ask if a specific assignment involving an art task will be helpful in increasing understanding of a particular issue. Some areas of clinical work can just as easily be explored through verbal means; for example, the concrete dimensions of laws, regulations and documentation are topics that are best discussed or read about through assigned readings rather than art making. In contrast, exploring the complexities of client-therapist relationships which involve emotional reactions, experiential work can often provide multilevel information, in addition to cut-and-dry facts not always accessible through verbal means.

One important area of concern in the use of art experientials within the supervisory session is the overlap of supervision versus therapy. Since most experiential art processes assigned in the classroom or supervision seminar are similar to what clients would be assigned, there is the distinct danger that the boundaries between therapy and supervision will become blurred. It is important to remember that using art has both benefits and problems in this regard. The same qualities that make art expression a useful thing in therapy will also be useful in supervision: using metaphor to explore complex thoughts and feelings, in problem-solving and achieving insight. However, there is the innate tendency of art expression to bring emotions more quickly to the surface. This may or may not be useful for some supervisees, just as it is not always useful to all clients. Also, if a supervisor's goal for supervision involves more cognitive understanding than personal exploration, then art making may not be appropriate or always ideal.

On the other hand, learning to work with people, applying therapeutic techniques and developing a professional identity are areas that not only involve critical thinking and cognitive skills, but also feelings and reactions that are not always rational and may be intuitive and/or personal. Art making within the supervisory setting may be the optimal way to explore these multidimensional aspects within a modality that is obviously attractive to individuals with an existing interest or passion for art expression. Wix (1995) also observes that clinical internships can be a particularly difficult time in the growth and development of art therapy trainees. She notes that it is a period when personal art making is often neglected while the student struggles with developing a clinical identity as an art therapist. The infusion of the art process within training becomes even more important at this critical time of developing a personal philosophy of art therapy in the workplace (i.e. practicum).

Lastly, using art making indiscriminately or in lieu of other ways of learning can be counterproductive. Some students may be actually resistant to using art making in supervision as they have often had a great deal of experiential learning in previous coursework. I can recall quite vividly a moment in a supervision seminar, when as supervisees we rebelled against the supervisor's request to draw yet another picture of something to do with 'our internships'. Although we all liked to make art outside the supervision session, it seemed to us that what we needed in supervision was some concrete information on what to do with clients at our various sites (and perhaps needed to rebel, as Riley describes in the evolution of the supervisory relationship in Chapter 3). The overall caveat is that one needs to be careful in the use of art experiences within the framework of supervision, constantly reassessing the assignment of art tasks according to the changing individual and/or group needs.

## Traditional Uses of Art Expression in Supervision

In the informal survey discussed in Chapter One, when asked "what methods do you use in supervision", approximately half of the respondents indicated that art making was a method they used at some time in supervision (the two highest ranked items were verbal discussion and case presentation).

However, from this small sample it is hard to say exactly how many supervisors use art making as a part of supervision and to what extent. Although the use of experiential assignments is common to both art therapy education and supervision, there has been little published on the topic. General concepts concerning the interface of art making and supervision have been discussed in a few papers by art therapists: art making and journal writing (Durkin, Perach, Ramseyer, & Sontag, 1989; countertransference (Fish, 1989); an internship studio (Wix, 1995). Considering the widespread use of art experientials within the training of art therapists, it is surprising that there has not been more mention of this topic.

In the field of counseling, there has been some interest in using art tasks to enhance supervision. Amundson (1988) notes the use of drawings by counselor trainees of their clients and counselor-client relationships and observes that they are useful in summarizing views about clients, providing additional insights and encouraging supervisory discussion. In a related article, Ishiyama (1998) developed a model for visual processing of client cases presented in counseling supervisory sessions. Ishiyama uses McKim's (1972) three basic steps of visual thinking (graphic ideation, idea-generation, and idea expression through drawing) to generate the following method of visually processing a client case: 1) describing the case in nonvisual terms; 2) generating metaphors and images for the purpose of conceptualization; and 3) drawing the case (1988, p. 154). The last step may also be completed through collage or a three-dimensional media of the trainee's choice. The process that follows these three steps involves presentation of the image to a group supervisory session where the supervisors and other trainees may provide feedback and share reactions to the art expression.

Since there is so little published on the use of art making in supervision, there is no data to support its use as having a significantly positive effect on the training or supervision of art therapists. However, despite the lack of research and understanding in this area, art making continues to be used by educators and supervisors with trainees and there is an apparent belief that art making is useful to some degree within the training process.

## Applications of Art Making to Supervision

Most uses of art expression in supervision have paralleled the use of art therapy with clients. In general, some type of directive is given and the supervisee visually explores the subject through art making using various media, assigned by the supervisor or chosen by the trainee.

There are a variety of simple directives that I have used throughout the years with both students and supervisees within graduate and postgraduate training. I am sure others have used these or similar activities, so the reader must excuse the lack of specific references to these ideas since they have emerged from the oral history of the art therapy profession. A few of the 'usual suspects' include:

- draw the client
- draw pictures of ideal and not-ideal clients at your site (see Fish, 1989, for related issues of countertransference)
- draw how you think the client sees you as the therapist
- make an image of the agency/internship site (to gain perspective on the dynamics)
- draw your experience of termination with a client or an internship site.

Visual journals have also been popular assignments and, in many ways, may be the most helpful (see Durkin, Perach, Ramseyer, & Sontag, 1989). Keeping a record of images along with some written thoughts throughout the internship experience is useful in not only recording reactions to the experience, but also in serving as a record of change and development. Some supervisors may prefer to review the content of the journals periodically in order to give the student feedback on the imagery. Sometimes visual journals become a series of not-fully formed images rather than a deep exploration through well-considered visual language. If this is so, it is important to clarify with trainees the depth of both imagery and exploration expected.

In order for a directive to be at all meaningful, it obviously must be used with care and respect, and more importantly contain a metaphor to explore through art. Therefore, although it may be easier to assign a specific directive to a group of trainees, the directive may not be useful to all members of the group at the time it is given. For example, to assign that the group make pictures of authority figures (see directive described below) may not be of particular interest or help to the trainees who have already explored and come to some resolution about this issue.

The display and sharing of art created to bring into group supervision sessions is another consideration. Everyone, including the supervisor, may be quick to jump to suggestions, interpretations and conclusions about the trainee's art and what it says about the trainee's potentials and problems as a therapist. These reactions may not be beneficial or wise in all circumstances. Being able to witness the work with a sense of objectivity may be the most helpful, thus respecting the very tender place that many novice supervisee's are in with regard to their work with clients and their own developing identities. Often, just letting the trainee tell the story of his or her art will bring up enough ideas and questions for discussion. If art therapists believe that much of the learning and growth in art therapy goes on during the art process, then a great deal of understanding will take place in a carefully chosen and defined visual assignment and sensitive witnessing of the resultant image.

Again, since the art assignment is not about personal therapy per se, then the treatment of the art expression should not be as one would treat art created in therapy. A trainee is an individual who is on the way to becoming a professional and is thus working toward independence and autonomy. Part of assigning an art project to a supervisee involves reinforcing the idea that learning through art making can be helpful to self-understanding and self-reflection, something that the supervisee will eventually need to do for him or herself when training is complete. Eventually the therapists-in-training must have the skills to self-reflect and explore the complexities of clinical work on their own and the supervisor should be cognizant of this goal when assigning art tasks to them.

## Some Additional Ideas for Experiential Work

The following directives are some I have used within either group or individual supervisory sessions:

**Authority figure:** This assignment is simply to create an image of an authority figure (see Figure 1). It is generally a group assignment with three people in each group working together to define the meaning of authority, conceptualizing the images, and finally creating a full size portrait on large paper. I usually offer chalk pastels and multimedia material(paper, magazine images, string, found objects) to create the image. The assignment can also be given as an individual exercise depending on the needs of the group or the goals of supervision.

The concept of authority is obviously a loaded issue and one that is not clearly negative or positive. Most people understand that authority in society (e.g. government, police, laws) is necessary to create safety and order so that we can function efficiently. However, there is a negative or ambivalent side that emerges when the idea of authority is brought up that involves misuse of power, control over others and imbalance. In Jungian terms, an authority figure can possess many qualities of the shadow aspects of humankind. Since authority is such a powerful archetype, the creation of a life-size figure will generate the most action and often some degree of acting-out. I have seen students sit supplicant beneath their life-size authority figure, others admire it and still others speak to it with words of hatred and disdain. One group of students even took theirs out and burned it! The image generates many diverse ideas, all of which are potent and charged but important to explore with trainees who are often struggling with authority at their practicum sites or jobs.

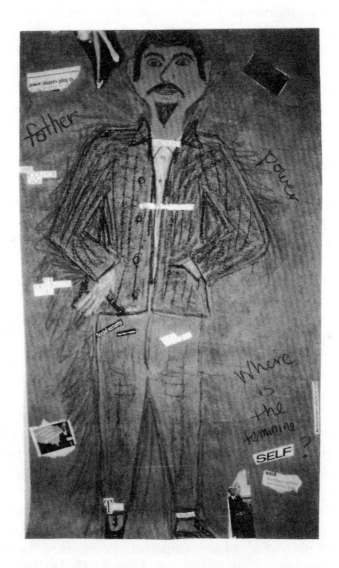

**Figure 1:** Authority figure created by master's level students

I originally developed this idea for work with clients in domestically violent or abusive relationships as a metaphor for power and control since an authority figure may very well be a perpetrator or someone who exerts power over another. I have also found it to be a particularly good exercise with adolescents who are often struggling with authority figures and their own issues of identity and independence. This developmental aspect of the process is important to remember, since many trainees are in the midst of their own 'adolescent' phase (see Chapter 3) of professional growth. Supervisees may be ready to attack authority and the supervisor who uses this exercise is forewarned that some adolescent acting-out may result from the experience. Also, since many art therapy trainees are female, there may be some additional issues related to abuse, harassment, and hierarchy that emerge from this assignment.

Despite the charged aspects of this process, it is an interesting metaphor and well-worth exploring in supervision. One of the major roadblocks to maturing into a professional is difficulty with authority or authority figures. This authority can be the practicum or internship site, an agency or facility, an administrator, an instructor, or of course, a supervisor. Authority can also be present in an abstract sense in the rules, regulations and structures that guide behavior and conduct. The identity of the therapist is tied to the concept of authority since therapists are considered by their clients as having a certain degree of power—perhaps the power to affect change or even heal. In this sense, the image a trainee creates of authority can be reflective of the struggle of assuming authority over others.

**Creating an Image of Supervision:** This assignment can be posed in a number of different ways depending on the situation, goals, and/or level of bravery of the supervisor assigning the task. You can ask the trainee any of the following: 1) how do you see supervision; 2) what would you like to get from supervision; or 3) how do you see the supervisor. The type of media can be left open although collage, drawing or simple construction seem to work well.

There are obviously many important and powerful issues that can be explored through this simple assignment. Since the ideal supervisor is defined by some as an individual who is empathetic, concerned, flexible, curious, attentive and understanding (Carifio & Hess, 1987; Holloway, 1995), the contents of an art expression involving this issue may happily meet these standards or may show that the supervisor has entirely missed the mark. In the case of the latter, the supervisor must be prepared for the soul-searching necessary to understand and deal with the uncomplimentary image presented by the trainee who may be underscoring some serious deficits or may simply

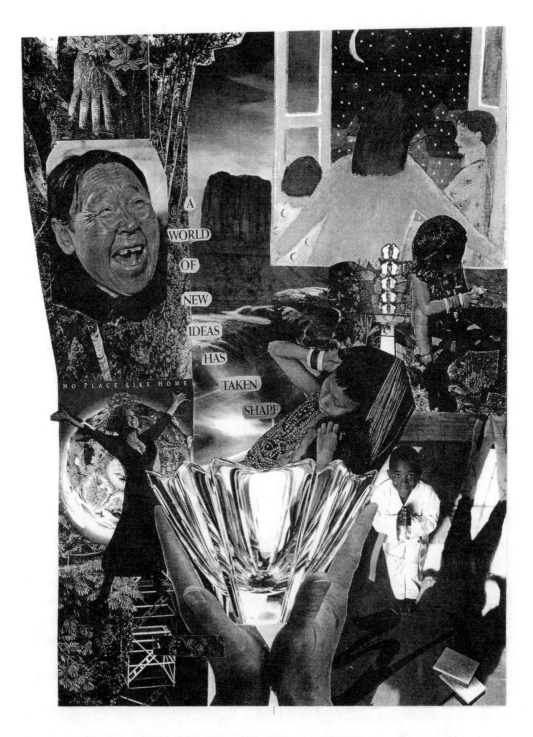

**Figure 2:** Image of supervision

be poking playfully at the supervisor's role of authority.

In Figure 2, a supervisee identified me as somewhat of a nurturer, a guardian and also a cohort (e.g. two birds of a different color). I recognized the common relationship of nurturer, caretaker and protector early on in the supervisory relationship. Since this intern was a few months from completing training, I was also pleased to see the cohort role evolving (i.e. two birds of similar style and color). I assigned the same supervisee the task of creating an image of 'what you would like to get from supervision' (Figure 3). The exercise was not only good for her and her explorations of her internship sites, but also gave me the feedback to know better how I could truly be of service to her in her development as a professional.

**Cartoon Strip:** This assignment involves developing a cartoon strip within a group (although it could be adjusted to an individual situation) by first creating a series of cartoon characters. The characters can be created by individual members of the group, but the assignment can be more dynamic by having each member draw one feature (e.g. eyes, nose, mouth, etc.) on a sheet of paper and then pass it to the person next him or her, who in turn draws another feature. This is done until a set of characters is completed, often appearing quite outrageous (Figure 4) and comical.

These characters form the cast of cartoon figures that eventually make up the cartoon strip. The next part of the process can either be open-ended (e.g. using the characters to create a spontaneous six-frame cartoon) or involve solving a situation or problem. Often I assign a problem to be addressed by the characters based on a theme that the group may be struggling with or want to explore further. In some cases, an open-ended approach is preferable but quite often a group needs a theme to guide them into confronting territory they might otherwise avoid. Often, by asking the group what they see as a problem or unanswered question will give the supervisor a direction for this activity.

This process is to a major degree, a way to problem solve, although there are obviously many other dimensions involved (e.g. who associates with what character or how the group works together). The idea was originated from working with pre-adolescents who developmentally find cartooning suited to their needs for caricature (Gardner, 1984). There may be a time within a trainee group that the supervisor observes the group to be developmentally at the pre-adolescent or adolescent stage, full of potential rebellion and wanting to poke fun at bosses, teachers, supervisors, a practicum site, a problem or a situation. Because they are in a rebellious mood, they may also be unfocused or anxious. Hence it is important to provide a more structured experience. The freedom and creativity in this exercise come from

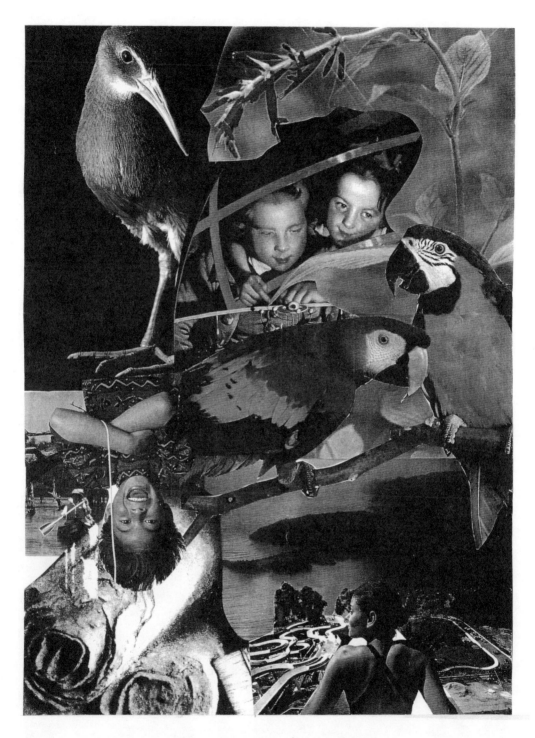

**Figure 3:** Image of supervision

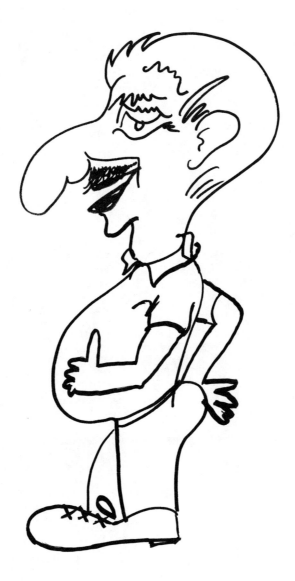

**Figure 4:** An example of a character for cartoon strip activity

the tradition of caricature drawing which allows features and characteristics of people to be drawn as outrageously as possible.

This process also encourages sequential problem-solving through the cartoon strip format and quickly generates interaction between group members, placing them in a situation of developing steps to achieve their goal or solution. Also, it often produces a variety of different solutions to the same problem. This is a trait which is intrinsic to critical thinking about therapeutic interventions and client treatment.

I have seen myself turn up in a couple of cartoon strips, once as a sort of saviour or ultimate guardian who protects supervisees from danger (Figure 5, the carnivorous cat who devours any threats to the trainees) and other times as a more reasonable sort of influence, benign but watchful. As in the previous directive to create an image of supervision, a supervisor may find a personal portrait of her or himself and be surprised at the characteristics of that portraiture. In this activity, by including caricature which is often graphically outrageous, the results may be even more surprising.

**Creating an Image of Professional Identity:** One of the long-term goals of supervision, particularly within graduate level training, is to assist students in the exploration and development of an identity as a therapist. Often supervision sessions are used by students to sort out ideas, theories, and ways of working with clients in order to discover what styles resonate with their own personal philosophies. Although the development and evolution of professional identity is a lifelong process, a major part of the development takes place within training and shortly after graduation, both times when supervision can help trainees sort out their confusion.

This assignment can be as simple or as complex as the supervisor would like to make it. A simple drawing or collage can be assigned; however, I prefer this be a long-term assignment that involves creating either a large image or even mask and costume of the professional identity. The assignment also includes writing about the image after it has been completed. Figure 6 is one of many examples of this exercise. This person's interpretation took the form of a mask of a wise old man—an image related to the supervisee's grandfather and father who were important influences throughout her life. About the image she writes:

> "When I think about being an art therapist, the basic image of healer to me is an 'old man'. This old man is not necessarily intellectual or knowledgeable. He is warm and caring. He is also genuine, playful and childlike. He knows both the pain and joy of growth.
>
> In my childhood, my healer was a grandfather who loved and took care of

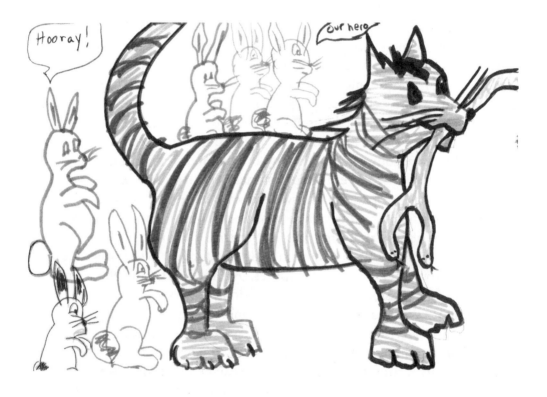

**Figure 5:** Cartoon strip showing supervisor as a carnivorous cat who protects the trainees from danger

me, taking the place of my busy mother. He had a magic hand with which he healed my aches and pains. The second professional model I have is my father, a doctor of medicine. He has been taking care of his patients for over 30 years and I see him as an older, healing man.

> Through this image I see myself working as an art therapist in many settings such as hospitals, clinics, nursing homes, and schools. I will be carrying the archetype of an old man inside me as a symbol of healing energy."

This is an appropriate exercise at the end of training or when a synthesis of ideas involving identity is needed. In a group supervisory seminar it can be a very powerful conclusion to the practicum experience and also very dramatic. Because the exercise can be quite involved, it should be assigned several weeks before it is to be presented in supervision to allow for reflection and in-depth exploration of ideas and images.

## Conclusion

This chapter has presented a few of the numerous directions that art making can take within the supervisory relationship. Since the purpose of art therapy supervision is to train art therapists, it is natural that art making will play some part in supervisory sessions. However, whether using art expression within the framework of supervision is helpful to learning remains to be seen. Ishiyama (1988) notes that there may be at least one possible drawback:

> "...there is a tendency of case presenters to become more self-focused than client-focused when the visual method is used. This is because generating metaphors and drawing cases are highly subjective processes... It is self-involving (for trainees) to place themselves and their subjectivity in the case drawings. Trainees' unfinished feelings, inner conflicts, anxiety, or self-doubt about their own competence as counselor may come to the foreground, and case presentations may turn into trainees' self-exploration. This itself may be highly meaningful, educational, and appropriate in supervision sessions. It may, however, be rather inappropriate or distracting in more objective and client-focused case presentations and discussions." (pp. 159-160)

This again underscores the point that the use of art making may be perceived as personal therapy, thus confusing the overall purpose of supervision (i.e. trainee's focus on client welfare) with one of solely personal exploration. It is reasonable to assume that personal exploration of feelings and conflicts about clients is important to successful supervision. However, it may become a delicate balance when art making, which can quickly bring emotional content to the surface, is relied upon for a large part of the supervisory experience.

Lastly, with the variety of materials and issues to be explored within supervisory sessions, it may seem difficult and time-consuming to some supervisors to infuse the art process into it. However, when used thoughtfully

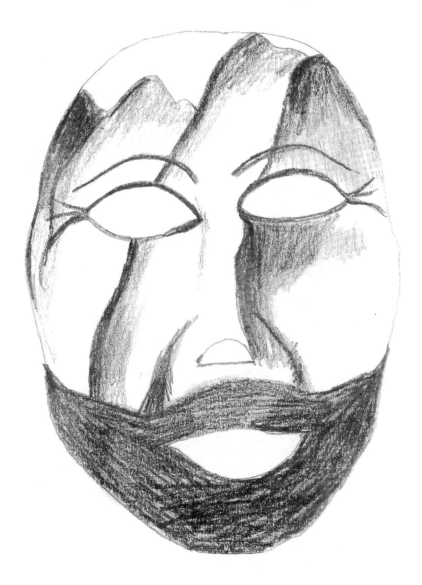

**Figure 6:** An image of professional identity

and strategically within a supervision group or supervisory relationship, there is no doubt that art expression can effectively enhance a trainee's development as a therapist, their understanding of clients and their personal reactions to practicum experiences. The inclusion of art making in supervision also underscores the rationale for using art as intervention through experiential learning and direct participation and more importantly helps to preserve the trainee's self-image as an art therapist. For these reasons, art making will certainly continue to have a place in many art therapy supervision settings.

## References

Amundson, N. E. (1988). The use of metaphor and drawings in case conceptualization. *Journal of Counseling and Development, 66,* 391-393.

Carifio, M.S., & Hess, A.K. (1987). Who is the ideal supervisor? *Professional Psychology: Research and Practice, 3,* 244-250.

Durkin, J., Perach, D., Ramseyer, J., & Sontag, E. (1989). A model for art therapy supervision enhanced through art making and journal writing. In H. Wadeson, J.Durkin, & D.Perach (Eds.), *Advances in Art Therapy* (pp. 390-431). New York: Wiley.

Fish, B. (1989). Addressing countertransference through image making. In H. Wadeson, J.Durkin, & D.Perach (Eds.), *Advances in Art Therapy* (pp. 376-389). New York: Wiley.

Gardner, H. (1984). *Artful scribbles.* New York: Basic Books.

Holloway, E. (1995). *Clinical supervision: A systems approach.* Thousand Oaks, CA: Sage.

Ishiyama, F.I. (1988). A model of visual case processing using metaphors and drawings. *Counselor Education & Supervision, 28* (6), 153-161.

McKim, R.H. (1972). *Experiences in visual thinking.* Monterey, CA: Brooks/Cole.

Rogers, C. (1957). Training individuals to engage in the therapeutic process. In C.R. Strother (Ed.), *Psychology and Mental Health* (pp. 72-96). Washington, DC: American Psychological Association.

Wix, L. (1995). The Intern Studio: A pilot study. *Art Therapy: Journal of the American Art Therapy Association, 12*(3), 175-178.

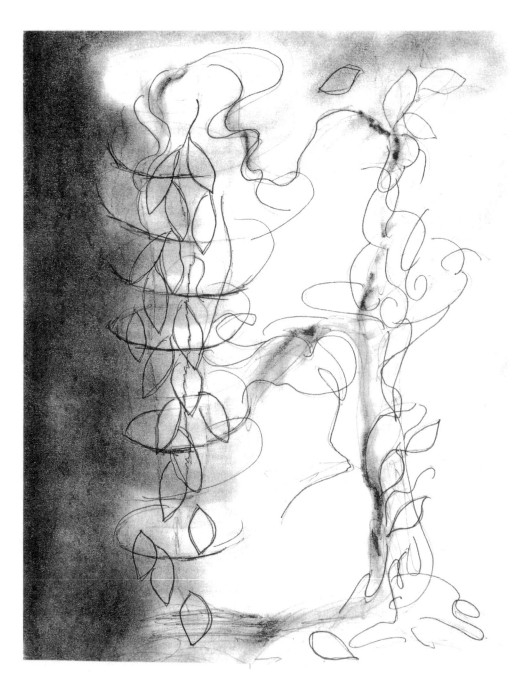

Supervision... reciprocal energy... setting the unique rhythm for each situation.

# CHAPTER SEVEN

## Peer Supervision
by Cathy A. Malchiodi

Peer supervision is recommended for therapists at all levels of development (Borders, 1991), but is rarely formally discussed. It can be loosely defined as both sharing professional experiences with other therapists in the field and providing specific advice or consultation to colleagues who may request it from you. It is probably the least well-defined type of supervision since it can occur on both a formal, contractual level, but more often occurs on an informal, casual level. Peer supervision may involve a small group of trainees or novice practitioners and an advanced practitioner who facilitates the meetings, or may be a group of peer practitioners who decide to get together on a weekly basis for collegial exchange. The former arrangement often includes a contractual agreement with the facilitator for a specific number of meetings listing the responsibilities of both the supervisor and supervisees. The latter is very informal, often with a verbal agreement among the members to meet on a regular basis to share client cases, discuss professional issues, or provide support and advice.

Peer supervision groups offer a forum for expression of ideas, feelings and concerns that can provide reassurance that one is having experiences similar to others. Most importantly, however, they can provide a forum for continued professional growth. For art therapists and other clinicians who use experiential modalities in their clinical work, peer consultation can provide the special focus needed to explore a specialized dimension of that work not easily available elsewhere. It also addresses the isolation experienced by many art therapists who may not have a peer colleague at their place of employment.

In a related vein, peer supervision may also be helpful to art therapists who may lose touch with others in their profession immediately after they leave graduate school. After formal training is completed novice clinicians often feel isolated and disconnected from the very field that they were extremely active in through their studies, practicum/internship, and research. Finding or forming a peer supervision group or at least locating a peer professional to have informal exchanges with, about case material and professional issues can help to reduce some of this sense of isolation and apprehension often experienced immediately after graduation.

Peer supervision groups serve a variety of purposes and are particularly diverse in the field of art therapy. Often professionals get together to share clinical material and methodology. Some peer groups have been formed for the purpose of making art or sharing creative writing as opposed to comparing clinical experiences. These groups may serve as an anchor for finding time for and receiving feedback on creative endeavors that are sometimes not a part of the work life of the individual. Other peer supervision groups may be composed of a diverse group of professionals such as social workers, psychologists, art therapists, etc. People may gather around a common approach (e.g. narrative therapy), a common place of work (e.g. the same agency or school), or a common interest (women's studies).

## Guidelines for Peer Supervision

Although many therapists participate in some form of peer supervision, relatively little has been written on this type of supervision, particularly group models (Borders, 1991; Spice & Spice, 1976; Wagner & Smith, 1979). This probably reflects the lack of literature on group supervision in general. Some of the most important goals of a peer supervision structure are: 1) inclusion of all group members in the supervision process; 2) maintenance of a common focus; 3) assisting members in giving each other objective feedback; and 4) a similar developmental level among members of the group. The potential for meeting these goals may be limited, given the composition of the group, the availability of group members and dynamics among members. For example, objective feedback may be difficult among a group of longtime friends or individuals who are overly concerned with hurting each other's feelings through providing constructive criticism. Additionally, members of the group may be at various levels of experience (e.g. novice and various degrees of advanced professionals), making a common focus difficult because of the multilevel needs of the members.

It is important to note that peer group meetings are not always helpful or productive (Borders, 1991), especially if goals are not established and adhered to (Roth, 1986), or if the members mainly give each other advice (Roth, 1986; Runkel & Hackney, 1982). Additionally, leaderless groups (which are common among peers) may have a problem staying on a central focus or keeping to a schedule of presentation and discussion. Over the years I have heard many peer supervision groups report the deterioration of the group due to an inability to retain a common focus, changes in group membership, or a general shift in the group members' interests.

In order to keep peer supervision groups on track, a designated leader or shared leadership among group members may be helpful. A leader (even if a different person assumes the leadership position from week to week) serves the important function of moderating the group and keeping everyone on track. He or she designates roles for group members, ensures that everyone is heard, and summarizes feedback. However, even with a leader or facilitator in place, the group may still eventually deteriorate.

To minimize some of the problems inherent to peer supervision groups, Borders (1991) advocates a structured approach:

> "The structured peer group approach provides the procedure and tasks needed for groups to capitalize on the benefits of peer feedback. The approach also offers counselors methods and skills they can adapt for consultative supervision with other counselors in their work settings and for self-supervision. By using approaches such as this one, counselors can actively contribute to their own professional development and that of their colleagues." (p. 248)

The approach Borders outlines includes several strategies which may or may not be applicable to all peer supervision but is specific to counseling. The author suggests including case presentation of client material (actually video tape of a session), followed by observations and feedback from peers. A designated supervisor facilitates discussion and summarizes the groups' feedback. A designated supervisor is considered by Borders to be the key factor in keeping the group on track and meeting the goals of peer supervisory sessions. However, an established protocol for each meeting is also necessary for the group to maintain its pace and structure.

Art therapists or those wishing to discuss art therapy interventions or professional issues may not find this approach meets their needs, particularly if supervision of clinical cases is not what they want. Instead they may wish to develop a structure for discussion of topics of common interest, readings, or viewing art (client or therapist). Art therapists may add the unique dimension of art making or sharing their own art within a peer consultation setting. Depending on the size and needs of the group, there may be a set schedule for presentation or responsibility for leadership/facilitation or it may be renegotiated when the group finds it necessary.

## Informal Peer Supervision

Many art therapists engage in some level of informal peer supervision without even knowing it. Since there are relatively few art therapists, it is not uncommon for one to reach for the phone to contact a colleague for advice or moral support. Others may get together at local symposia, conferences and chapter business meetings with the purpose of professional enrichment, but end up spending a great deal of time talking about therapeutic strategies, agency politics, association politics, dilemmas and struggles with the art therapist's identity. This often occurs at the national conference level where advanced professionals seek each other out, hungry for support and collegial discussion of topics pertinent to their practice or area of interest. As art therapy increases in recognition and more people seek training, I have found myself getting calls from other countries, too, where trainees and professionals are basically looking for advice, consultation, and mentorship. Some of these individuals are professionals in other disciplines, but have had some level of art therapy training and simply want to connect with another professional for suggestions and direction.

During graduate school students often form peer groups outside the classroom or clinical supervisory sessions to get support or exchange ideas about methodology and practice (or about a difficult professor or supervisor!) Although these types of sessions cannot replace the advanced and knowledgeable supervision a master clinician or instructor can provide, they can and do establish group communication and set the stage for future networking when the students have graduated and joined the professional ranks as therapists.

## Ethical Responsibility & Peer Supervision

As with any type of supervisory experience, ethical responsibility is an important consideration. When there is one clearly defined facilitator or group leader, well-delineated goals, and regularly established meetings, it is easier to develop a contract concerning the accountability of both the group leader (the supervisor) and the members (supervisees). This is similar to any other type of supervisor/supervisee relationship, although the purpose of a peer supervision group may be more specific (e.g. have a particular theme or goals) than other types of supervision groups. Therefore, any guidelines, laws, and ethics that govern the conduct of supervision are applicable.

In other circumstances, however, peer supervision may be much more informal and it may be more difficult to address the issue of accountability.

In a loosely structured group of peer colleagues, there may be no formal rules or goals beyond the purpose of providing support for each other's work. There are usually no formal contracts created among group members that address responsibility, leaving open the possibility of problems in the areas of ethics and accountability.

Depending on the nature of the group (e.g. a group which discusses case material versus a book or journal club), there may or may not be legal or ethical concerns. One legal issue may be the sharing within a group, client material which is considered confidential (a more in-depth discussion of confidentiality is presented in Chapter 13). In any case, ground rules for what can and cannot be discussed outside the group are important to establish at the outset, if only to reinforce personal and professional ethics. Additionally, if one of the group members appears to be violating an ethical code or regulation, what are your responsibilities as a member of the group? This question and others that come up may not be easy to answer, given the informal quality of most peer consultation. However, questions concerning accountability may arise especially when case material is exchanged and other group members provide feedback and suggestions. Lastly, dual relationships can also be a potential problem, since peers are often friends and, as friends, know and share personal details and confidences.

## Suggested Guidelines for Peer Supervision Groups

Although there are a variety of aspects to consider when forming a peer supervision group, here are some basic suggestions for structuring a group for art therapists:

1) Set a time each month to get together (or at regular intervals).

2) If possible, try to include group members with similar caliber, professional stature, and training to reduce developmental differences.

3) Decide how to structure the time you spend together: e.g. will you each take turns presenting a case, will it be a journal or book club where everyone reads the same material for discussion, will you get together to make art and discuss it, will each one present a new technique or approach each meeting, etc.

4) Consider having a group leader or taking turns at leadership. For novice professionals, it may be wise from the outset to either contract with a more advanced professional to be the supervisor/leader. Art therapists with several or more years experience may want to setup a leaderless group format; however, they should establish clearly from the start the need to stay with the group's goals and purpose of the peer supervision.

5) Consider what the group is responsible for in the area of ethics,

particularly confidentiality, and how the issue of accountability will be handled within the group.

## Cyberspace: Peer Supervision in a Post-Modern World

Having spent a good deal of my professional life in a sparsely populated western state, there were times not so long ago that I was the only art therapist in the region. Even today there are only a couple of professionals in my field that I can call if I need to talk to another art therapist and some of these folks are in neighboring states. There are still many areas of the United States (and the world) where there still are not many art therapists, particularly those with advanced training in the field.

Luckily, post-modern technology has made it easier for those who are geographically isolated to communicate with others around the country and even around the world. The advent of cyberspace and on-line communication has greatly enhanced everyone's ability to network quickly and easily with people that were previously inaccessible (except at prohibitive cost by telephone). In *The Saturated Self* (1989) Gergen describes the post-modern phenomenon of cyberspace:

> "Electronic mail first served those mainly within one city or organization. Most large cities offer bulletin-board services, which allow individuals to place an announcement of their interests on a file open to all users of the system. In this way computer conversations develop, and fanciful subcultures spring to life, sharing interests—any time of day or night—in areas ranging from African art to aphrodisiacs, backgammon to banjos... There is almost always 'someone' there to talk to... Many participants speak of the warm and accepting relationships that develop within these context—much like the corner bar, where there are always old buddies and new friends." (p. 59)

Another related development is the advent of virtual reality, allowing one to encounter events and experiences vicariously through computer technology. One wonders if the technology termed virtual reality could result in something we may someday call virtual supervision. It would be fascinating to put on a pair of virtual reality glasses and enter a program that would take you into virtual supervision within a scenario of working with a particular (virtual) client and also to have at your disposal an advanced (virtual) clinician who could give you virtual feedback on your virtual interventions or virtual therapeutic style.

That may be a few years away, but there are several venues available right now that somewhat echo the concept of virtual reality. An area of growth for peer supervision is the abundance of computer on-line opportunities for exchange with colleagues not only in one's field, but also experts in related professions literally throughout the world. The Internet and the newer World Wide Web (known as the Web and WWW) have a variety of formats for professional exchange, the most well-known being 'newsgroups' that cover specific areas of interest. There are also Web pages that can be accessed through on-line topic searches similar to exploring a library computer database; once accessed, an individual can find more specific information on the topic or leave messages for the Web page sponsor.

In order to enter cyberspace, one simply needs a computer with an appropriate amount of memory, a modem (a device which connects the computer to an existing phone line), and computer program or on-line service that allows access to cyberspace. Computer on-line services include Compuserve, Prodigy, Genie, and America Online, four of the most familiar ones with others surfacing all the time. Each service offers direct access to the Internet and the Web as well as specialized forums for users to exchange ideas and make connections with other professionals. For example, for mental health professionals there are currently on-line opportunities to interact with marriage and family therapists, psychologists, social workers, and medical professionals, among others, through bulletin boards and newsgroups where messages can be posted or through live, on-line events where people can chat with each other by typing in responses and opinions. Topics in on-line newsgroups, message areas, and discussion groups vary from day to day, but it is fairly easy to make a request for information or develop a discussion on a topic of one's clinical interest.

There are also opportunities to learn about other related areas such as legal issues, ethical issues and professional writing as well as easy connection to databases with research and current information. I have regularly participated in forums on marriage and family therapy, alternative health, and medicine, topics which are specifically related to my private practice and consulting services. I also get involved in the occasional writers' forum to help me hone my skills as an editor and writer, and art forums to give me a chance to converse about the arts. One can tailor on-line involvement to what is needed at a given moment and easily locate information and feedback in a variety of diverse areas of learning, often within a single on-line session.

On-line message areas are not only excellent places to connect with other professionals in a peer setting, but they are also particularly good for learning more about client populations as well as various trends and current methodologies. For example, over the last year I have participated in on-line cancer support groups where people discuss their feelings about having cancer or being a caregiver of someone who has a life-threatening illness. This experience enhanced my understanding of cancer clients in ways that would have otherwise taken months of time and research. Also, a request that I made for information about working with AIDS clients generated several helpful messages as to where to locate information and several bibliographies on working with this population.

On-line mini-conferences (often called chat or discussion groups) are another avenue for communication and are scheduled regularly, often with predetermined topics. Through these conversations, I can interact with people throughout the country simultaneously, learning what someone who lives in New York, California, or Ohio thinks or experiences, without leaving my home office (and even in my favorite bathrobe!) to travel some distance to a site. If you live in an area where there are very few art therapists, on-line conversations can be a literal lifeline to find out instantaneously what others are thinking and doing in diverse parts of the country. On the Internet and the Web the exchanges can be even more far-reaching; one can regularly hear from professionals in Europe, South Africa, and Australia via electronic mail and in some cases, live on-line events.

A colleague, Barbara Levy, MPS, A.T.R.-BC, and I started a folder for creative arts therapists in late 1994 on the America Online service. After a few weeks of us just talking to each other, the word got out and more colleagues joined in the exchange. By mid-December we were able to host an on-line mini-conference to discuss issues of interest to the group. By the following year the list of those participating had grown considerably and the dialogue had matured to include issues of governmental affairs and licensure, private practice, surviving managed care and changes in health service delivery. It reaffirmed not only my belief that colleagues in the field are eager for professional exchange, but also that the cyberspace format provided accessibility to a diverse group of individuals. Additionally, the forum provided a voice to a group of professionals and students across the United States who might not be able to come to annual conferences to share ideas and receive face-to-face feedback.

Again, some words of caution are necessary when participating in on-line exchanges, particularly concerning clinical discussions. Whatever you type onto your computer screen for transmission to a newsgroup, on-line folder, or download will be available to anyone who visits that area. It can be copied and distributed elsewhere without your knowledge or permission. Since the Internet, the Web, and on-line services have no copyright standards, everything that appears on them may be used by others, somewhat like public domain. If you send a private message to another colleague, realize also that what you say is in writing just like a letter or any other document. Computer on-line forums are informal ways to connect with other professionals but you may not always get the advice and answers you are seeking. On the other hand, the opportunity for unrestricted exchange and interdisciplinary networking is limitless and is increasing as more and more people come on-line.

## Conclusion

This very brief chapter touches on some of the issues involved in peer supervision. If anything, peer supervision is a way to stay connected to one's professional field and to enjoy communication and exchange with one's colleagues. It is also a valuable resource for therapists throughout their careers, offering support, debate, and discussion necessary to stay current in one's thinking and practice. By engaging in peer supervision, either formally or informally, therapists can contribute not only to their own professional development, but also the development and enrichment of their colleagues.

---

Note: Any of the following computer on-line services offer connections to the Internet, the Web, newsgroups, and live chats: America Online, Compuserve, Genie, and Prodigy. Other software programs, such as Netscape, are available to allow you to send and receive e-mail or gain access to the Internet and World Wide Web. Because status of these services changes so rapidly, you are advised to consult software catalogues and magazines on computer products for the latest information.

## References

Borders, L.D. (1991). A systematic approach to peer group supervision. *Journal of Counseling & Development, 69,* 248-252.

Gergen, K. (1991). *The saturated self: Dilemmas of identity in contemporary life.* New York: Basic Books.

Roth, S. (1986). Peer supervision in the community mental health center: An analysis and critique. *The Clinical Supervisor, 4,* 159-168.

Runkel, T, & Hackney, H. (1982). Counselor peer supervision: A model and a challenge. *The Personnel and Guidance Journal, 61,* 113-115.

Spice, C., & Spice, W. (1976). A triadic method of supervision in the training of counselors and counseling supervisors. *Counselor Education and Supervision, 15,* 251-258.

Wagner, C., & Smith, J. (1979). Peer supervision: Toward more effective training. *Counselor Education and Supervision, 18,* 288-293.

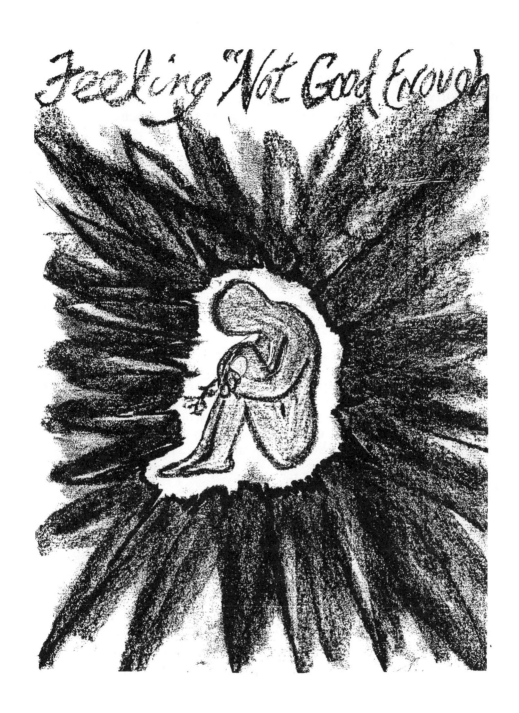

# Feeling Not Good Enough

A flower emerging... the hope for future competence.

# CHAPTER EIGHT

## Supervising Supervisors
by Shirley Riley

This chapter will focus on an area of supervision that is undefined and to my knowledge, rarely written about: the supervision of supervisors. It is a form of supervision that is used and encouraged in many training programs as well as other environments. Placement coordinators in academic programs often supervise the supervisors in the field, who supervise the student-trainees in practicum. Another situation that calls for this form of supervision involves private practice where a supervisor asks for individual or group supervision to consult about specific problems. These settings have commonalties and differences that I will address and, in addition, propose the need for establishing standards and structures for art therapists who have been designated to, or who choose to take on this responsibility.

One professional organization that specifically addresses the role of the supervisor of supervisors is the American Association of Marriage and Family Therapists (AAMFT) which has developed detailed standards for supervision. The AAMFT publication, Supervision Bulletin of the American Association of Marriage and Family Therapists, discusses current issues in supervision and is sent to 'Approved Supervisors' of the AAMFT as part of their yearly fees to maintain that status. Although this bulletin is published by a family therapy association, the material it contains is universal for all disciplines that involve supervision. The American Counseling Association (ACA) has developed similar standards for supervisors and has a division, the Association for Counselor Education and Supervision (ACES), which focuses on training and supervisory roles of counselors. Both the AAMFT and the ACA/ACES guidelines are important documents to review by those who intend to supervise either trainees or other supervisors.

There are also some articles written about essential fundamentals that are the basis of supervision and should be read by those who wish to supervise other supervisors: Sluzki (1974) on the usefulness of the isomorphism concept; Liddle (1988) on conceptualizing the goals of supervision; Haley (1976) on factors in selecting a training context; Berger and Damman (1982) on the supervisor's multidimensional vision of supervisory techniques; Edwards (1994) on 'reflection' as an important component of supervision; Fienberg (1993) on ethical and practical issues in supervision; and Durkin, Perach, Ramseyer, & Sontag (1989) on a model of supervision enhanced by artmaking. These and other articles listed in the references of the chapters in this text contribute to the body of knowledge that the advanced supervisor brings to the task of supervising supervisors.

## Caveats for Supervisors of Supervisors

The supervisor of supervisors may overlook the fact that in addition to providing advanced supervision, they also become libel in the chain of ethical behaviors involved in legal actions (see Chapters 13 & 14). Therefore, if you choose to be a supervisor of supervisors, it is of primary important to examine your malpractice insurance policy and be sure that you are covered for all the actions of the persons involved in this supervisory sequence. It is also important to make sure that the supervisees are well-insured. It is necessary to be protected, since problem situations that may be presented in supervision could be legally challenging.

If problems arise, outside agencies and social services may be affected and other professionals will have vested interests in their interpretation of the clinical difficulties. I am thinking in particular of cases of abuse where the parents have been confronted with neglect and the child, or other member of the family, has been removed. Often the therapist is expected to continue treatment with all or at least segments of the family. To proceed with therapy under these conditions, be it with the family or an individual, raises many questions and places the therapist in a paradoxical position (even more so, if they have reported the abuse and 'caused' the disruption in the system, and are still supposed to be trusted by the clients). How the "Supervisor" consults with the supervisor, who then advises the therapist, who then conducts the therapy, becomes a chain of actions that may result in a number of outcomes. Some may be very threatening to all involved. This example shows how vulnerable each of the participants of this relationship may become. In a litigious society, it becomes obvious that to be unprotected is not an option. Yet many of us take on the supervisory role without thinking of these possible consequences.

Another general concern is one that involves competence. If a supervisor agrees to advise another supervisor, what criteria of expertise should they expect of one another? In the field of healthcare, professionals who do not have standards for supervision (such as the AATA at this writing) it becomes a personal decision as to what each party expects from the other. It seems essential and obvious that a supervisor must have experience and competencies in the field of healthcare in which they supervise. The supervisor they request for additional supervision should have greater expertise and experience, but by who's criteria and with what guarantees?

I suggest that common practice be the guide and that we turn to the other fields of health care to find the accepted standards. For example, the Board of Behavioral Sciences which is the licensing agency for the State of California, insists that no credit for supervision is accepted unless that supervisor has been licensed for a minimum of two years. This seems like a reasonable time frame that could be translated for art therapists to two years (or more) after receiving Art Therapy Registration (A.T.R.). The supervisor of supervisors should, in my opinion, have an additional five to eight years of experience as a supervisor to qualify as a supervisor of supervisors.

It appears that we must monitor our own supervisory relationships at this time, but I imagine it would be natural to seek out someone who has demonstrated superior skills to be one's mentor. Just as I would imagine that to accept a mentorship, one would hesitate to consult and advise with a person who had prematurely placed themselves in the responsible position of supervisor without adequate experience. The specter of legal action and loss of practice may, unfortunately, be a deciding and motivating factor at this time.

McNiff (1986) describes the excellent clinical supervisor in this manner:

"The excellent clinical supervisor is self-confident and possesses diversified theoretical and practical knowledge of the creative arts therapies as well as the principles of various psychotherapeutic systems, has the respect of colleagues within the clinical setting and the ability to clearly articulate the clinic's orientation to professional practice, is flexible and adaptive to the differing needs of students, is empathetic and able to transcend personal perspectives, encourages students to allow their unique qualities and therapeutic styles to emerge, has a sophisticated self-understanding and is aware how personal behavior affects others, does not insist upon a single theoretical model for therapy, is able to clearly articulate what is happening within the supervisory relationship and when necessary confronts problems, inspires the students with standards of quality, provides both professional and personal support and affirmation, assists in the resolution of ambiguity while maintaining respect for the complexities of clinical practice, and helps the student to integrate theory and personal values with therapeutic practice." (p. 159)

This discourse demonstrates the multitude of themes that must be woven together to complete the fabric of supervision.

## Common Hazards

The conduct most often breached in supervision is that of entering into a dual relationship with the supervisee (in this chapter's focus, the supervisor-in-training). It is wise to give a clear definition of this hazard to the supervisors that are being supervised, particularly, since it is not uncommon for those therapists that are seeking supervision to be colleagues, previous students of the supervisor, or fellow professionals from the workplace. The alliance is clouded from the start with the shadow of past connections (see Chapter 13 on Ethics).

The balance of clear boundaries between two supervisors, within a learning situation, not only keeps the interactions where they belong (on the client), but also is a reflective experience that is passed on to the trainees by example. In other areas of shared experience with clients and in the workplace, the collegial approach and a more egalitarian attitude toward advancing the knowledge of clinical exploration, makes supervising supervisors exciting and rewarding. However, if the relationship slides toward the parameters of therapy the novice supervisor may not be aware of the contamination, and makes it a model that will be used with their interns in the future. Like a malfunctioning family script, it is passed from generation to generation.

The supervisor seeking supervision should look carefully into the philosophical stance of the supervisor he or she chooses in regard to their practice of art therapy. There are conflicting views on the use of visual expression in clinical work and this remains a sensitive area that is unique to our field. For example, if a person has a strong belief in the open studio opportunity for participants, it would be problematic to engage the services of a supervisor who does not agree with this approach and prefers structured assessment procedures to dominate the course of art therapy. There are many conflicts around the use of art, the frequency of it's use, the advantages or disadvantages of a variety of procedures, and it's integration with theory. It becomes incumbent on the supervisor requesting the services of the advanced supervisor to explore all these issues and more. The art therapy is the heart of the process and must be the center of the supervisory agreement. This does not rule out choosing to explore a variety of ways of achieving the art therapy experience, but to be at basic odds with the reality of conducting art therapy makes for unneeded tension in the supervisory relationship.

## Supervising Supervisors in an Academic Setting

In my experience the task of supervising supervisors that are supervising the student/trainees in their practicum, falls on the Placement Coordinator (PC). This person is usually a faculty person and may function in several roles. The PC either arranges for the placement of the students in practicum or approves the practicum site that the students find for themselves. In both cases the trainee should have on-site supervision by an accredited staff member, (i.e.) a licensed clinician. In addition, the art therapy intern must have supervision by a registered art therapist who may be on site or off site. The students' appointment to the practicum and the contractual relationship with the supervisors, both clinical and art therapy, should come through the school and be part of the students security in their education. There are some cases where the student must seek and pay for their own supervision. In this case there can be very little control exercised over supervision and the student is less protected. In all cases the supervisor of the supervisors has multiple goals in this multi-leveled association. The PC acts as liaison between the agencies, the school, and the trainee. S/he must mediate in conflicts between any component of the above mentioned system. Her first duty is to support the student, and second, attend to the supervision or agency demands that have disrupted the training opportunity. The aspect of mediation should be a skill taught to the supervisors in the field and can be the focus of a discussion group with the supervisors.

Within the academic purview the supervisory issues may be addressed through regular supervisors' meetings; scheduled by the school and mandated that the supervisors attend (depending on the policy of the school). The meetings should be interesting enough that the supervisors feel that they are gaining information and advancing their understanding of the specialty of supervising. Successful therapists who dedicate their time to supervision usually have a busy life. We cannot expect them to give up their precious time to attend meetings unless they gain more than just the prestige of being named supervisor.

If the school provides basic training for supervisors before they enter into the supervisory position, it enhances the cohesion of the group. A course serves another purpose by bringing the new supervisor in line with other more experienced clinicians, giving the supervisor (placement coordinator) a more unified audience with which to work (see Chapter 9, Course of Study for Supervisors). The supervisors' meetings can be handled in many ways, however, the basic goal is to familiarize the supervisors with the present philosophy of the program. Inviting special speakers that are able to talk about current thinking in the field is a stimulating reward. The faculty could, on occasion, discuss the evolution of the program and enhance, in that way, the supervisors' feeling of belonging to a team effort. Their suggestions and feedback can be influential in bringing the academic program into the real world of mental health needs.

Problems with students may be discussed if confidentiality is preserved. If a problem is discussed, it should be slanted toward how the issue can be prevented or solved, not on a personal level. Video presentations of key dilemmas in supervision can be very revealing. Encouraging students to video their sessions is an important issue and taking videos of supervision with a trainee can inform them both about parallel process and the clinical conduct of the art therapy session. If these tapes are shared in meetings with the supervisors, a lively form of the reflective team technique can help the supervisor to evaluate a supervisory relationship and the methods of teaching and learning. This is a stimulating addition to supervision.

As art therapy practitioners enter the field, they come with a basic body of knowledge gained through the masters program, their own supervision, further experience, and some continuing education. It is how continuously this last item has been pursued that causes concern. Too often the pressures of job and family have given the art therapist an excuse to stay within familiar boundaries of practice, and as the mental health and educational world moves ahead, they do not. Therefore, there is an unevenness in the practice of therapy, the practice of supervision, and the education of students-in-the-field. Regular meetings of the supervisors can counter this deficiency. This is the most efficient way for the supervisor from the program to supervise the supervisors and encourage commonality of good practice.

## Supervising a Supervisor in Private Practice or as an Independent Contractor

If a supervisor requests supervision outside of the structure of the university, the considerations are quite different. The one requesting the supervision is the one in control and the advanced supervisor becomes the provider. Therefore, establishing goals, time frames and financial arrangements are issues that must be discussed immediately. Often the supervision is geared toward achieving compentence in a particular area or working for a certificate or acquiring acknowledgment in the field of supervision. The practice of video-taping sessions of supervision with their interns is one of the best resources for ongoing assessment. The intimate check and balance system within a university system, with student evaluations and feedback, and information from agencies, is not available in private practice. Instead, the training must be more intensely focused on the actual use of techniques and understandings of the process of art therapy and the dialogue created between the two supervisors engaged in this contract. There should be assigned reading in the field of supervision and an additional written component, with the goal being to enlarge the scope of the supervision. In some cases the one being supervised will be unwilling to assume these extra tasks and the advanced supervisor must then weigh how her/his supervision will be used. If it is for personal growth alone, then the requirements can be flexible. If the supervision requires written evaluation or a letter of approval at the completion of the time period, then a more considered attitude must be taken and greater investment made in the educational component. The approving supervisor is risking his/her reputation by attesting to the competence of another supervisor.

Caution and consideration must be the guidelines for giving professional approval. The supervision should be able to confirm: 1) the content and skills that were demonstrated for supervision, 2) the methodology used, 3) the theoretical base from which the training stemmed, 4) the setting and population where the supervision took place, and 5) their form and method of evaluation. This material should be supported by videotapes demonstrating competencies from the above areas.

## Summary

In any setting, formal training program or informal personal contract, the final goal is the same. The supervisor must be able to conceptualize and clarify the goals of supervision. Supervision is a context in which different levels of learning occur and the supervisor must have a multidimensional vision of supervision (Berger & Dammann, 1982). Supervision provides an arena where contrasting experiences can exist for both participants and a training experience where the thinking is changed for both parties (Ibid). If the supervisor of supervisors has succeeded in raising the level of awareness of the complications and potentials both for growth and diminution that are built into the supervisory relationship, then much has been accomplished. Skilled supervision is a resource that has been acknowledged as one of the greatest opportunities for increasing therapeutic skills and educating the novice therapist. However, the quality control factor has been sadly neglected. There is room for stimulating examination of this field and an untapped opportunity for art therapists in particular, to find unique ways to improve the level of supervision. Since no hard rules have been put into place at this time, there is a chance to change our system to include the proven strengths of other training approaches and introduce individual techniques and goals that are appropriate for the art therapists' ways of working.

## References

Berger, M., & Damman, C. (1982) Live supervision as context, treatment, and training. *Family Process, 21,* 197-205.

Durkin,J., Perach, D., Ramseyer, J., & Sontag, E. (1989). A model for art therapy supervision enhanced through art making and journal writing. In H. Wadeson, J.Durkin, & D.Perach (Eds.), *Advances in Art Therapy* (pp. 390-431). New York: Wiley.

Edwards, D. (1994). On reflection: A note on supervision. *Inscape, 1* (1), 23-27.

Fineberg, M. (1993). Training art therapy students to be supervisors: ethical and practical issues. *American Journal of Art Therapy, 31*(2),.109-112.

Haley, J. (1976). Problems of training therapists. In J. Haley (Ed.) *Problem-Solving Therapy* (pp. 169-194). San Francisco. Jossey-Bass.

Haley, J. (1988). Reflections on therapy supervision. In H. Liddle, D. Breulin, & R. Schwartz (Eds.), *Handbook of family and marital therapy* (pp. 358-367). New York. Guilford Press.

Liddle, H., Breulin,D., Schwartz, R. & Constantine, J. (1988). Training family therapy supervisors: Issues of content, form and context. *Journal of Marital and Family Therapy. 10,* 139-150.

McNiff, S. (1986). Educating the creative arts therapist.Springfield, IL: Charles C Thomas.

Sluzki, C. (1974). Treatment, training, and research. *Unpublished paper presented at the Ackerman Memorial Conference in Venezuela.*

## Also see:

*The Supervision Bulletin:* Information concerning American Association for Marriage and Family Therapy Approved Supervisors. Washington. D.C.: AAMFT.

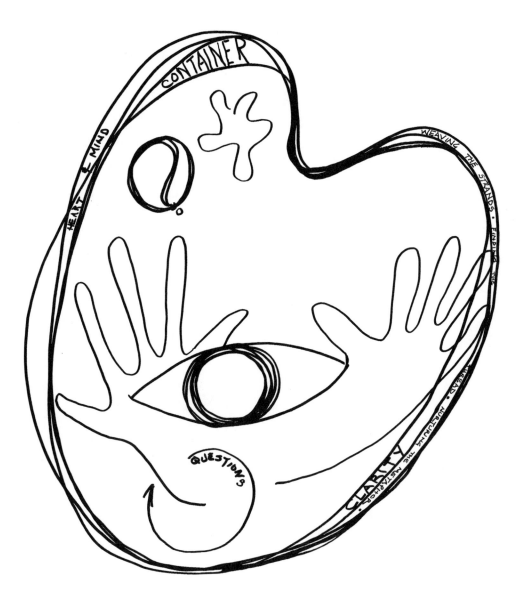

Supervision: Seeing and supporting, a container for questions,
finding the way, weaving the metaphor.

# CHAPTER NINE

## A Course of Study: Training the Art Therapy Supervisor
by Shirley Riley

    This chapter offers a course designed to train art therapy supervisors within academic programs or agencies and institutions. The author supports the notion that the course be offered within an established educational setting. However, it is not enough just to present the itinerary, as outlined below, to aspiring supervisors; the supervisor/educator/instructor must be capable of addressing individual situations as they arise and have the ability to conceptualize and teach the principles of supervision. Additionally, the attendee should research and be satisfied with the credentials and experience of the supervisor teaching the course.

    The course of study outlines six three-hour classes providing training for therapists to become qualified supervisors. The objective is to educate students in the basic skills of supervision. The instructor should be a Registered Art Therapist (also licensed, if necessary to fulfill state or other regulations) with a minimum of five years of supervising trainees, interns, and/or colleagues. It is recommended that the instructor be an experienced teacher, be well-read in the field of supervision, and be able to include additional material in the outline if the situation so requires.

    To qualify for the course the participants must meet the standards required to fulfill the role of future supervisor. Suggested qualifications for therapists to enroll in this course are: 1) s/he be a registered art therapist with at least two years, postmasters degree, clinical experience; 2) s/he has received personal supervision; and 3) any other requirements which state or national organizations have delineated as necessary background experience (see Chapter 2, for suggested standards for supervisors).

Each member of the class must present a video of themselves working with client(s) and explain the process of the session in context and in theory. A reflective team will act as supervisors of the session and discuss the process with the presenter. This videotape is a requirement before the participant in the class may receive the certificate of completion of the course.

Three texts are recommended for this course; additional reading or articles should be added to meet the specific needs of a specialized program or population.

**Recommended Texts:**

1. Kaslow, F. (1986). *Supervision and Training; Models, Dilemmas, and Challenges.* New York: Haworth.

2. Hess, A. (1980). *Psychotherapy Supervision.* New York: John Wiley & Sons.

3. Malchiodi, C., & Riley, S. (1996). *Supervision and Related Issues: A Handbook for Professionals.* Chicago, IL: Magnolia Street Publishers.

## Course Outline

### Class One: Beginnings - *Focus on the Supervisee*
How to establish the structure, boundaries, time, and place of supervision

—Discuss the supervisee's responsibilities regarding; 1) clinical case documentation; 2) presentation of the client art work and protection of the client's art product; 3) establishment of clinical goals; and 4) preparation for the supervision hour with questions for the supervisor.

—Discuss the format of supervision: 1) the supervisory relationship and its' limitations; 2) the concept of dual relations and the need for therapy outside the supervision; 3) the legal responsibility the supervisor carries for the intern's clients; and 4) the need for malpractice insurance.

—Explore students' common fears and expectations of: 1) supervision in general; 2) their immediate supervisor; 3) the agency and the administration; 4) the client population; and 5) the supervisor's expectations of their performance.

—Assign readings of ethical documents.

It is important to note that ethical issues are not confined only to the beginning of the supervisory relationship, but are ongoing concerns that may be returned to at any time in the course or as warranted. It is also recommended that an emphasis be placed on teaching the "evolution" theory of supervisee's growth and a tolerance for individual learning styles of the participants during the first class meeting.

An art experiential may conclude this first class and should be structured to invite the novice supervisor to recall his/her own past experiences as a new supervisee. This could be a "memory" drawing, followed by a dialogue: "What was positive and what was difficult in your first phase of supervision?" The question can also be raised: "Do the members of the class feel that supervision would have been improved if their supervisor had been trained for the responsibility?"

**Recommended reading for Class One:**

1. In Kaslow, *Development of Professional Identity in Psychotherapists; Six Stages in Supervision Process*, Friedman & Kaslow, Chapter 3.

2. In Hess, *The Transition from Supervisee to Supervisor*, Styczynski, Chapter 3.

3. In Malchiodi & Riley, *The Evolution of the Supervisory Relationship*, Riley, Chapter 3.

4. In Malchiodi & Riley, *Art Therapy Supervision: An Overview*, Malchiodi, Chapter 1.

5. In Malchiodi & Riley, *Documentation & Case Presentations*, Malchiodi, Chapter 11.

6. In Malchiodi & Riley, *Exposure and the Consequences of Legal Liability in Art Therapy Training & Supervision*, Kollar, Chapter 14.

## Class Two: Development - *Focus on the Supervisor*
Explore the tasks of the supervisor

—Articulate the supervisor's theoretical belief system and process of integrating art therapy in the treatment; check the current curriculum in which the program trainees are enrolled, or inquire about the dominant theoretical attitude of the agency or practice where the supervisee works.

—Establish confidentiality concerning supervision, the clients clinical material, the art work, and the evaluations.

—Encourage an open dialogue about the success and failures experienced by the supervisee in the client sessions.

—Question the transferential reactions in supervision and in the client relationship.

—Study the parallel process between client, therapist, and supervisor.

—Examine supervisory boundaries: supervision is not therapy.

A role-play with the class may be devised that reflects their questions concerning one or more of the issues referred to above. The script of the role-play can be extrapolated from an actual case being seen by one of the class members if confidentiality is maintained. If there is no material from the class, the instructor will provide a situation that challenges the supervisors-in-training to solve a problematic situation (e.g. recognizing a dual relationship).

**Recommended Reading for Class Two:**

1. In Hess, *Psychotherapy Supervision and the Duality of Experience*, Barnat, Chapter 5.

2. In Hess, *The Dilemmas of Supervision in Dynamic Supervision*, Rioch, Chapter 6.

3. In Kaslow, *What Do Therapists Worry About: A Tool for Experiential Therapists*, Charney, Chapter 2.

4. In Kaslow, *Growth in Supervision: Stages of Supervisee and Supervisor Development*, Hess, Chapter 4.

5. In Malchiodi & Riley, *Clinical Issues Related to Supervision*, Riley, Chapter 2.

6. In Malchiodi & Riley, *Exposure and the Consequences of Legal Liability in Art Therapy Training & Supervision*, Kollar, Chapter 14.

## Class Three: Re-experiencing Media

—The class will be experiential and is designed to broaden the attendees' use of a variety of media and rekindle an exploratory approach to the art therapy process.

—Share new or previously used media that evoked successful outcomes in therapy; try these approaches in the class.

—Speculate when (or if) the traditional or experimental use of media may advance or hinder therapeutic process.

—Discuss the limitations that agencies impose on the art therapist; purchasing media, small budgets, room crunch, lack of storage, the mysterious loss of media (sometimes by clients and sometimes by fellow workers); how to handle this loss; how the supervisors have solved some of these problems; Does the use of art set you apart in the agency? To your benefit? To your depreciation?

—Reminders about the potential danger of using toxic or sharp tools in the art session.

During class draw an image related to one of the issues that are a challenge in providing supervision, or draw "your supervisory relationship with your supervisee". After using one media to express one of the challenges referred to above, change the media and reflect if this changes the meaning of the product.

**Recommended Reading for Class Three:**
1. In Malchiodi & Riley, *Integrating the Art Process in to Supervision*, Malchiodi, Chapter 6.
2. Art therapy articles on media contributed by class members.

## Class Four: Focus on the Process - *Treatment & Goals*

—Discuss the various methods to observe if a supervisee is competently making the art therapy expression an integral part of the treatment.

—Discuss how to help the supervisee deal with the non-expressive client and how to resist a power struggle with the client who refuses to do art.

—Examine how the supervisor makes it clear that his/her expectations are that art therapy will be utilized in the majority of client session. Are there exceptions? Explain how the supervisor takes responsibility for bringing this subject into the supervision.

—Review how the supervisor can help the supervisee with assessment of the client and the continuing necessity for assessment; discuss the variable methods of evaluating the progress of the therapy.

—Explore how the art therapy process moves the treatment toward the desired goals: the need to consider "fitting" the therapy to the context of treatment. Appraisal of the best approach for individual, family, or group treatment.

—Reflect on the best way to retain focus on the goals of treatment and still remain flexible when approaching these goals.

—Discuss the use of video observation, the use of audiotapes, and the presentation of the client art work to clarify the achievement of goals.

—Consider the belief systems of the client, the supervisee, and the supervisor to better protect the supervisory relationship from being contaminated by personal and biased judgments.

The exercise for this class meeting would involve small groups engaging in a role-play (with prepared scripts) that forces the therapist to set treatment goals with the client. For example, divide the class into several small groups and give a child-focused symptom situation to one group, an adolescent group task to another and a family crisis case to a third. The learning will be slanted toward the recognition that the process and goal achievement must be structured differently in each case.

**Recommended Reading for Class Four:**
1. In Kaslow, *The ABCX Model-Implications for Supervision*, Sharon, Chapter 5.
2. In Kaslow, *Themes and Patterns*, Chapter 14.
3. In Hess, *Vertical Supervision*, Glenwick & Stevens, Chapter 17.

4. In Malchiodi & Riley, *Videotape Recording in Supervision & Live Supervision*, Riley, Chapter 10.

## Class Five: Focus on the extended systems - *Social and cultural pressures in treatment*

—Introduce the importance of looking at social issues, such as violence and unrest in the community, in the media, and in the client's environment. How do these external circumstances influence treatment and the effective conduct of therapy by the supervisee?

—Discuss the radical change in the value system between generations, between designated class levels, between the urban and rural societies and the impact on the art therapy treatment. Has it changed the imagery? Can supervisors and supervisees read the art through their lens if they differ economically or socially from their clients?

—Explore if the image can be understood if the language of the metaphor is foreign to the therapist.

—Explore how the supervisee, together with the supervisor, can be constantly alert to bias and differences.

—Examine how supervisors can help the supervisee to de-pathologize clients by looking first at their external stressors and life threatening events, before giving a diagnosis.

—Touch on the issue of case management and its place in treatment.

This class could be enriched by guest speakers with expertise concerning various cultural world views and literature that explain a variety of cultural/ethnic values. Art tasks that encourage the class members to externalize their own prejudice and become aware of their unresolved attitudes toward a group(s) could also be used. Small group discussion structured to challenge denied prejudice is recommended.

**Recommended Reading for Class Five:**

1. In Hess, *Racial, Ethnic, and Social Class Considerations in Psychotherapy Supervision*, Gardner, Chapter 29.

2. In Hess, *Supervision in Community Settings: Concepts, Methods, and Issues*, Aponte & Lyons, Chapter 25.

3. Articles from current journals that reflect on this ever changing issue in society, brought in by instructor and class members.

## Class Six: Focus on Gender Issues and Contemporary Attitudes

—Review how the current status of women, men, gay and lesbian issues are reflected in therapy.

—Discuss if these gender issues have been considered in art therapy literature. Has there been any preferred method of treatment that takes these vital facts into consideration? Discuss if it is possible for a supervisee (or anyone) to understand another person's gender experience.

—Explore the issue of power in gender defined roles, in class defined roles, in the role of therapist vis a vis the client. Look at the issue of power in the supervisory relationship.

—Explain how the theories of psychotherapy may conflict with the current interpretation of equality, in gender, in role assignments, and in the position of the therapist.

—Does the gender of the supervisee and the supervisor (if not the same) have any influence on the therapeutic relationship? How can the supervisee best deal with sexual issues, sexual overtures and harassment, which could be encountered in client treatment or in supervision?

—Discuss how to help the supervisee find therapeutic art directives or strategies that will address these sensitive issues.

—Help the new supervisor with ways to open up discussion around their own difficulties in this gender defined domain and how to resist becoming a therapist to the supervisee when these issues are discussed.

—Invite discussion of problem areas, particularly if there are differences between the supervisor and supervisee in gender, in race, in age, in social class, etc.

The art task for this class meeting could focus on the conflicts of gender assigned positions in society or families and bring them into focus through the imagery. It would be appropriate to use material from social issues exploited in the media to demonstrate how these pressures impact the gender issue.

**Recommended Reading for Class Six:**
1. In Kaslow, *Themes and Patterns*, Chapter 14.
2. Additional articles contributed by class and instructor.

## Overall Recommendations for the Course:

Each class should be at least three or four hours, allowing the flexibility for didactic and experiential material as well as informal discussion.

Each class would benefit from engaging in an art process that externalizes some of the clinical issues or experiences the supervisors have encountered recently. This is an important opportunity for the class to deepen their involvement in the supervisory process.

Time should also be given for the participants in the class to bring up individual difficulties or successes they recall in relation to supervision or related issues.

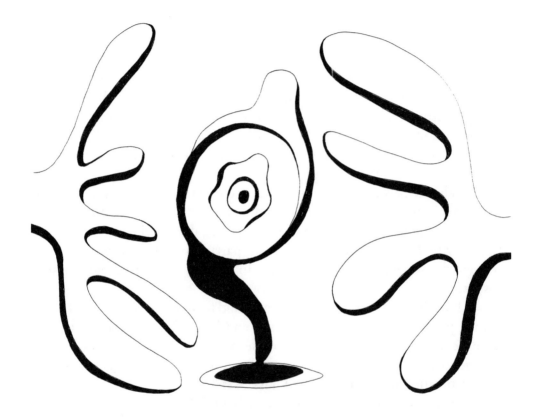

Supervision feels like a supportive environment to explore and receive clarity about artwork... we reach toward understanding the art from all sides. As we search together for understanding, the art takes on a life of its own and seems to evolve in our presence.

# CHAPTER TEN

## Videotape Recording in Supervision & Live Supervision
by Shirley Riley

This chapter will demonstrate the many benefits to be gained by the use of videotaping in the process of art therapy supervision. Not only does the visual record add depth to the shared understanding of the treatment under discussion, but the in vivo observation of the content and context of the session provides greater opportunities for support and helpful criticism. This tool also eliminates misinformation and misunderstanding in clinical reporting.

Videotape recording is particularly useful in art therapy supervision. A therapy that honors the power of the image and the creative process is a therapeutic service that identifies with visual communication. Therefore, supervision should also incorporate a visual approach. An art therapy session with an individual client, a family, or a group must be seen to be fully understood. Art therapy is concerned with the product in the sense that it often contains material that comprises a metacommunication upon the issues at hand. However, it is often the process of the creation of the art that is essential to evaluating the worth and potential of the therapeutic contact.

When a supervisee brings client artwork to supervision and attempts to describe the process of the creation, it is not easy to get a sense of the timing, the pacing, or the affective mood sustained during the production of the work. These aspects are essential for the supervisor to understand and observe in order to guide the supervisee in conducting art therapy. The following discussion makes a case for the use of videotaping in supervision.

## Brief History of Live Supervision

Live supervision has been recognized as one of the most creative and practical mode of supervision in training novice therapists. The Philadelphia Child Guidance Clinic, under the precept of Salvador Minuchin and his colleagues (Colapinto, 1988), established the use of the one-way mirror in the training of laypersons and professionals guided by experienced therapists on staff. Suggestions to the therapists were telephoned to the session from behind the one-way mirror during the session and, when necessary, the treatment was interrupted by the therapist leaving the room for consultation.

Other schools of therapy continued in this tradition of the use of live supervision. For example, the Milan school used a team of four therapists, two with the family, and two behind the mirror (Pirotta & Cecchin, 1988). When the session was near completion, the four therapists consulted and then gave the family a prescription for further treatment based on their mutual decision. The MRI group in Palo Alto, CA also used this type of observation during their early work attending to communication and behavior patterns with the schizophrenic patients and their families (Fisch, 1982).

The complete division between the client(s) and the observers changed with the technique of the "Greek Chorus" practiced by Peggy Papp (1980). She introduced a greater freedom between consultation, observation and the participation of the client(s) in the session. Recently, there has been an even greater shift away from secrecy about what the observing team is thinking and doing. Andersen (1987) felt that the "reflecting team" could interact with persons in treatment and encourage an understanding of their interactions by directly sharing the team's evaluations. Eventually, Andersen discarded the mirror entirely and placed the clients in the same room with the team. They could either observe the therapist from behind the mirror or listen to their discussion of the session in the therapy office (Whiffen, 1982; Montalvo, 1992).

Many therapists became convinced that a reflective team was useful in supervision as well as in therapy. Hoffman (1993) has discussed how she uses reflective team principles regularly, both in training and in supervision. In writing about the reflecting formats, she has this to say:

> "They have transformed my supervision work, my teaching, my consulting, and my workshops. Due to the more horizontal relational structure I encourage, most of my groups turn into home-rooms where people can find emotional sustenance and a noncompetitive environment." (p. 160)

From this description we can see how the therapist came out from behind the mirror and into the co-creation of therapy with the client or family as well as in supervision. Many additional articles have been written about live supervision and the information is useful when considering ways to enrich the context of supervision (Haley, 1976; Hare-Mustin, 1976; Whitaker, 1976; Berger & Dammann, 1982).

In an interview recorded in 1992, Braulio Montalvo (the author of a classic paper on live supervision in 1972) has some additional thoughts about live supervision:

> "Live supervision should not be the only tool used in supervision but used with others. Supervisees learn different skills from what I call synoptic supervision—supervision in which supervisees summarize several of their therapy sessions with a case...It is the contrast between 'talking about' or abstracting from the 'raw stuff' and 'seeing in the real world' that provides supervisors with something to work on with their supervisees. Each method is a window to help supervisors and supervisees gain information and refine the tools of the therapist." (p. 1-2)

The use of live observation has not been as extensively discussed with individual treatment; however, it is just as effective when evaluating the course of therapy with an individual as with a family group. The examples mentioned above are not comprehensive and further reading can be found in the reference section at the end of this chapter

## The Introduction of Videotaped Supervision

As technical advances brought down the price of video cameras, videotaping replaced the one-way mirror in many clinics and teaching institutions. National conferences on therapy, for example, often videotape a master therapist working with a family or an individual in one room, and project the session simultaneously on a big screen in the convention hall. This is an opportunity for the observers to see "in vivo" the triumphs and mistakes made by these brave therapists. As a person who has personally experienced this exposure, I must say that it is a challenge that cannot be taken lightly. As White (1994) recently said "I am tired of being given the most difficult, impossible situations to solve in my demonstrations" (p. 42).

Nonetheless, the videotaped session is a very useful tool for both the therapist and the supervisor. Observing another therapist not only educates how he or she uses their approach, but also how personality commands theory. Goldenberg and Goldenberg (1991) offer this information:

> "According to Whiffen (1982) videotaping has three unique properties that make it especially valuable in supervision: 1) it freezes time so that every aspect and angle of a crucial sequence is available for post-therapy play and replay by the therapist, impossible to achieve during the session; 2) it enables the therapist to see himself or herself more objectively as a contributor to the whole system, a different perspective from the one in the midst of the often bewildering multiple stimuli

occurring during the session; and 3) it allows the effect of the therapeutic intervention to be studied and its success evaluated." (p. 298)

The videotaped hour has the advantage of permanence for several reasons. The therapist can review the tape carefully and gain a great deal of knowledge about the progression of the session, the achievement of the projected goals, the efficacy of the interventions and the changes in the client or family. The supervisor can spend time viewing and reviewing the tape with the supervisee. Also, the clients can see the tape with the therapist and add their evaluation to the understanding of the session. The clients, in particular, gain a sense of being more in control of solving their own problems and being a part of the therapeutic team rather than the object of discussion.

A video presentation captures the interactions in the session in an indelible way that allows the supervisee and supervisor the luxury of assessing the progress of the therapy more than once. A live session can be seen only the day it is scheduled, and if the supervisor misses that appointment it is gone forever. With videotaping there is never a 'lost' session. By viewing the videotape in supervision, the growth and continuity, both of the client and the supervisee, can be reinforced.

Videotaped supervision is desirable on all levels of the supervisory contract. It enhances learning and supports the relationship between supervisor and trainee. A successful intervention is never overlooked, difficulties can be appraised in context, and misunderstandings avoided.

## Questions Answered Better by Viewing the Therapy than by Reporting

A list of questions follow that could be the foundation for supervision and evaluation of a session observed through live or videotaped supervision:

1. What gave rise to the introduction of the art process?

2. Was the therapist attentive to the subtle signals from the client(s) that could have lead to a suggestion for the theme of a drawing (for example)?

3. How soon into the session did the trainee introduce the notion that using the art would enhance the goals articulated by the client?

4. Did the supervisee encourage verbal explanation of the art product?

5. Did the original creative activity follow a previous product; did it lead into further expression based on the material revealed in the art?

6. Did the therapist establish therapeutic goals that evolved from the transactions around the art product?

7. What satisfaction did the client experience from the use of the media? Did the therapist explore a variety of media with the client to enhance the production of the art?

These are only a few of the vital questions that should be considered in every session between supervisor and supervisee, including those sessions which are videotaped. This list of inquiries can be modified to fit the population and setting where the therapy takes place, as well as the level of sophistication of the supervisee's experience.

Looking at this list of questions makes it very clear that none of these processes can be clearly explained in a supervision session with only the verbal recall of the supervisee to convey the process. The supervisor may get an entirely wrong impression of the course of the contact with the client(s). This misinformation could lead to clinical advice that in turn will not be compatible with the best interests of either the client or the supervisee

## Resistance to the Use of Videotaping Art Therapy Sessions

The profession of art therapy has traditionally been reluctant to borrow techniques from other fields of mental health. There have been concerns expressed over the possible inhibition of creativity that may occur if the client is aware that he or she is being recorded by camera. In parallel reaction, the art therapist who has never, or rarely, been videotaped in session also is afraid that the spontaneity of the relationship might be diminished if recorded. The self-conscious discomfort of being observed the first time or two can only be counteracted by actually experiencing this form of observation. The resistance that new therapists anticipate is often a projection of their own anxieties.

The question of the client or family agreeing to videotaping has a great deal to do with the way the opportunity is presented to them. They should be informed in the first contact session that the therapy will be recorded. If the therapist explains that this is an opportunity for the clients to help the therapist understand their transactions more competently, they will become more involved in assessing their own patterns of behavior.

In addition, a release form is always offered to the clients and no taping can be done without the clients' permission. The clients should understand that they will be the ones to review the tape and that they have the right to eliminate any part of the video after they have seen it. It should be made clear to them that the tape will be used in supervision to insure the quality of their treatment. They may wish to meet the supervisor and that should be arranged. Since some clients may have taken videos of themselves at gatherings or holidays, they can be reminded that they are experienced subjects and that the therapist will need their help at times.

In a class I teach in the second year of a masters program in art therapy, a videotape of work with a family is required of students. Each student shows an edited portion of the tape to the class, which has been reviewed with their supervisor. The class acts as a reflective team, supporting his or her efforts and pointing out the strengths of the session. As the leader of the class I control any tendency toward abusive criticism. The students also write confidential comments to the presenter, to further enhance the opportunity for feedback. Without exception, when it is announced that a videotaped session is required, the class becomes agitated and worried. This distress is somewhat alleviated by role-playing the first session when the proposition of being taped is made to the family. However, in spite of the apprehension, the majority of the students report how quickly they, and the clients, forget about the camera. Sometimes the session is enhanced by the cameras being the focus of the therapy. The watching eye of the video may remind clients of the watchful eye of the parent, the neighbors, the welfare system or any number of authority or critical situations in their life. Often the camera brings out the "ham" in the clients, the children in particular, and there may be a few moments of acting before the session gets underway.

Another major advantage of students sharing their work in this manner is the support and comfort they derive from seeing that they all are beginners, that they all have "impossible" clients, and that in spite of their misgivings and anxieties, the clients profit from the art therapy treatment. Video recording can be seen as another aspect of the creative adventure with art therapy. At the end of the semester, the majority express this feeling: "I have never learned as much as I have from being forced to make this video. Watching it taught me more about myself as a therapist than I expected."

The following video evaluation can be given to the students to fill out and return to their classmates following the observation of the taped session presentation in class.

# VIDEO EVALUATION FORM

To further enhance the experience of making a videotape of a family session from your practicum, the class is requested to offer the presenter additional feedback. The following answers may be anonymous and will not be censored by the instructor. Each week all members of the class are requested (on the honor system) to give the previous week's presenter his or her respectful evaluation.

Please consider the following issues:

1. Were the goals of the therapy established early in the session?

2. Did the therapist stay on track and move the therapy forward?

3. As the art task became established did he or she display flexibility if the art task needed to be reconsidered? Restated?

4. Was the art "imposed" on the family, individual or group or did it emerge from the therapeutic dialogue?

5. Was there a summary of some kind at the conclusion of the session?

6. Did the art work receive sufficient attention? Exploration? Changes observed? Reflections made?

7. What personal mannerisms or techniques would you advise the therapist be sensitive to in the future?

8. Did the therapist pick up on metaphors that fit the family or individual? Reframe the behaviors with the goal of finding new meaning in established patterns?

9. Was there a feeling of trust and empathy present in the session?

10. What did you find exciting, interesting, informative, useful, challenging in this session?

## When Videotaping Is Not Useful

In spite of the advantage to the clients in observing how their interactions affect each other and the parallel learning opportunity in supervision, there are times that this technique is not acceptable or is counterproductive.

For example, an agency's policy may forbid videotaping of their clients under any circumstances. This has been circumvented, on occasion, if one shows only the back of the client, or keeps them off-camera except for their hands and art work. However, the intern cannot control the system and may have to accept the policies. A second instance is when the material is so sensitive that exposure of the tape would put the client at risk (for example, a sexually molested child revealing material around the abuse) and of course, the third block to this mode is the client who adamantly refuses to be on camera. No power struggle will aid the client in achieving their goals in treatment.

Therapists and supervisors may be convinced that videotaping is of great advantage to all involved, but they must be realistic about the settings where most new therapists get their training. In spite of the difficulties inherent in making a change in policy in hospitals and community mental health agencies, it is still important to persist in implementing videotaped sessions. When videotaping was first introduced at the university at which I teach about six years ago, the training sites were quite resistant to the idea. They were anxious about patient confidentiality and interruption of the therapeutic process. Over the years they have seen how careful the university is about release forms and, more importantly, how responsive the clients are to this amplification of their treatment.

## Supervising Supervisors by Videotape

Some professional organizations encourage the use of videotaped or live supervision in the training of supervisors. For example, the American Association of Marriage and Family Therapy (AAMFT) offers an "Approved Supervisor" recognition for persons who meet their standards for advanced training in supervision. The process requires, among other qualifications, eighteen hours of supervision by an AAMFT Approved Supervisor. The hours are videotapes or live observations of the supervisor supervising. The supervisor is put in the same position he or she has put their trainees. To be scrutinized by one's peer is slightly different, but the same anxieties may be present.

I recently had this experience and after many years of supervising and guiding supervisors in an academic program and in private practice, I wondered how I would profit. I did not doubt that I would learn a good deal, but what? My narcissistic person was somewhat fearful and also somewhat arrogant.

My insecure self was afraid of being exposed as inadequate. The surprise was that the process of being supervised after all these years and the learning through watching the tapes was a wonderful experience. I had forgotten how rewarding it is to be attended to for a concentrated period of time with the goal clearly articulated as a time for me to grow.

I learned a great deal about my stylistic quirks; some were just amusing and not harmful to the client or the supervisor, others were inhibiting to the supervisee in their search to find answers. My training supervisor pointed out times when I asked closed questions—questions that did not invite exploratory replies. I was unaware of this; however, I became much more attentive to this fault after seeing and hearing myself make this mistake. I saw myself 'lean into' the session when I was deeply involved, and 'lean out' of the session when I was ready to make an observation that was, perhaps, hard for the client(s) or supervisee to hear. That body language was totally unconscious. I had to spend some time thinking about the meaning of the rhythm, for myself and the supervisee. What message was I sending? I realized that I would have never had the opportunity to observe and then discuss this personal behavior if it had not been recorded on videotape.

At the completion of the required hours I was reluctant to terminate. I realized that I had not had this opportunity for self-growth in a long time. I concluded that all supervisors should have the pleasure of becoming a learner again. The same reaction that my students have after their videotape assignment is completed, I had the pleasure of experiencing myself.

## The Future of Videotape in Therapy and Supervision

There are many in the field of art therapy that would agree that supervisors would be making a mistake if our profession is not willing to experiment with this method of expanding the quality of supervision. It would be an opportunity to encourage an interchange between art therapists living at a distance from one another; to be able to ask advise from experts out of your area; and to share new, effective methods of teaching and performing therapy as well as supervision. Fear of the camera is widespread, but after a brief exposure to the lens the attention is on the client and the self-consciousness disappears. I hope this method of examining the process with another colleague will be the next step for most training and supervisory sites in the not too distant future.

## References
Andersen, T. (1987). The reflecting team: Dialogue and meta-dialogue in clinical work. *Family Process, 26* (4), 415-428.

Berger, M., & Dammann, C (1982). Live supervision as context, treatment, and training. *Family Process, 21* (3), 337-344.

Colapinto, J. (1988). Teaching the structural way, In H. Liddle, H., D. Bruelin, & R. Schwartz (Eds.), *Handbook of Family Therapy Training and Supervision* (p. 17-37). New York: The Guilford Press.

Fisch, R. (1988). Training in the brief therapy model. In H. Liddle, H., D. Bruelin, & R. Schwartz (Eds.), *Handbook of Family Therapy Training and Supervision. (p.* 78-92). New York: The Guilford Press.

Goldenberg, I., & Goldenberg, H. (1991). *Family therapy: An overview.* Pacific Grove, CA: Brooks/Cole Publishers.

Haley, J. (1976). *Problem solving therapy* .San Francisco: Jossey-Bass.

Hare-Mustin, R. (1976). Live supervision in psychotherapy. *Voices, 12,* 21-24.

Hoffman, L. (1993). *Exchanging voices.* London: H. Karnac.

Molvado, B. (1992). Live supervision as a window. *The American Association of Marriage and Family Therapy Supervision Bulletin, 5* (2), 1-2.

Papp, P. (1980). The Greek chorus and other techniques of paradoxical therapy, *Family Process, 19,*45-57

Pirotta, S, & Cecchin, G. (1988). The Milan training program. In H. Liddle, H., D. Bruelin, & R. Schwartz (Eds.), *Handbook of Family Therapy Training and Supervision* (p. 38-61). New York: The Guilford Press.

Whiffen, R. (1982). *The use of videotape in supervision: Recent developments in practice.* London: Academic Press.

Whitaker, C. (1976). Comment: Live supervision in psychotherapy. *Voices, 12,* 24-25.

White, M. (1994). Panning for gold. *The Family Therapy Networker, 18* (6), 40-49.

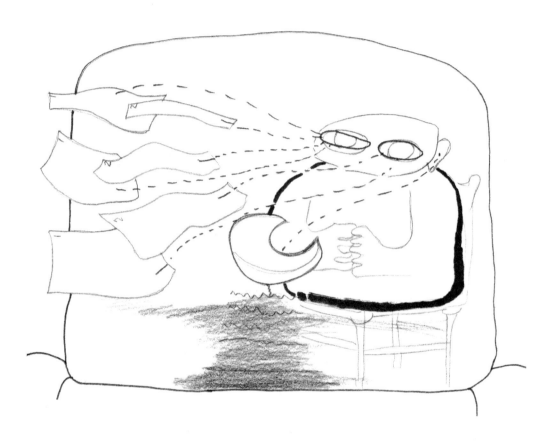

The paperwork! All I can see!

# CHAPTER ELEVEN

## Documentation & Case Presentations
by Cathy A. Malchiodi

Trainees often have many questions about documentation of their sessions with clients. Documentation can include many things: the use of clinical charting or progress notes as part of client's records; written observations assigned for practicum or internships; clinical or psychological reports; and written and oral case studies that are either part of a course or as a final project for a degree. Students, particularly first year graduate students with no previous clinical experiences, often have difficulties in initially learning to prepare notes and case materials on clients. Many trainees have been accustomed to writing about arts and humanities; more technical writing and documentation presents a new and challenging approach to organizing thoughts and ideas.

Also, some of the difficulty and confusion about documentation comes from the lack of information on how to specifically undertake writing about clients in both clinical and academic settings. Much of this mystification stems from the fact that no matter how careful and meticulous a therapist is about notes and observations, there is more or less always a subjective quality about them. However, there are ways to structure observations so that although they may be somewhat subjective, they follow a logical thought pattern and convey information clearly and professionally.

## Charting & Progress Notes

The term 'charting' comes from the day-to-day notes that clinicians are required to write concerning patient progress and treatment planning. It is a type of brief notation that is seen most often in hospital or clinic settings, and is used to record the contact that various clinicians have with a client, and the type, objectives and result of contact. In some settings a clinical supervisor must read and sign the supervisee's charting or progress notes. In all cases, a supervisor should be aware of a supervisee's ability to chart and record his/her interactions with the client and his/her understanding of different methods of charting.

General rules about charting and progress notes include: the date and time of day when the note is actually recorded; what kinds of notes were made (e.g. individual, group, family; regular session; special sessions such as consultations; summary, termination and/or referral); and listing of the problem or goal of the treatment. One very common method of charting is called SOAP; the letters are an abbreviation for the following areas of documentation:

**Subjective:** A subjective statement about the client.

**Objective:** The outcome sought for client (goals).

**Assessment:** The client's strengths and assets, liabilities or barriers to change. Brief comments on the client's progress toward goals that the therapist has set for him/her and a brief assessment of client statements and art expressions may be included here.

**Plan:** A description of the future plans for the client or continuation of current treatment goals. What is planned, when, and for how long? List specific interventions and methods, frequency of contacts and expectations for achievement.

In this age of managed care, the means and dates of evaluation are also important. Therefore, it is important to note how and when the progress of the client will be determined and evaluated. In a hospital setting this may take place within a treatment team, however, in any setting it is important to consider how the goals and treatment plans will achieve the desired outcomes on behalf of the client.

SOAP notes are intended to help the therapist and health care team plan a successful course of treatment for the client. Narrative notes are also used in some facilities instead of SOAP or other formats. There are several other charting methods besides SOAP; most of them are based on a medical model of notation and are behaviorally-oriented. For example, Zuckerman (1995) suggests the following simple format:

- Date of Plan
- Problems
- Goals in terms of behavior or actions to be changed
- Method, interventions, or actions to be used to achieve goals
- Results or outcomes desired

- Resources/strengths of client in achieving outcomes
- Target dates for completion of treatment and dates of reviews of plan.

Since record-keeping is accomplished differently at each agency or internship site, it is often best that the supervisor initially request that the supervisee bring in samples of the treatment plans, relevant forms and any other materials that will describe the requirements for notation. In hospitals and clinics, there are usually standard formats that are used and are readily available. On the other hand, in community or social service agencies there may be no formal charting per se and record-keeping may consist of minimal information or census data. For example, shelters for the homeless usually do not have the same system or level of charting that a hospital psychiatric unit does, since a shelter is not, by definition, a healthcare facility. Facilities for battered women and their children, which often see large numbers of individuals for short time periods, also do not keep the same types of client paperwork as more clinical milieus. In these situations the supervisor and supervisee may want to work out a system of client record-keeping that will satisfy the need for progress notes and also support the trainee's learning experiences in this area.

Since art therapy trainees are often exposed to several different practicum sites, it is important to understand and adapt documentation styles to the trainees' individual learning experiences throughout supervision. The practicum or internship site where the trainee is placed and the population that the trainee works with, will effect the type of record-keeping style needed. For example, a psychiatric hospital will require a different style of recording client progress than a classroom for learning disabled children. Notes recorded in schools may involve forms or narratives that will be part of a student's academic file and/or notes and summaries on Individual Educational Plans (IEPs). Or, in social service agencies such as shelters, halfway houses and crisis intervention agencies, case management styles of record-keeping may be used. Finally, the advent of managed care has brought with it new forms and specific ways to record client treatment plans, assessment data, and outcomes. Therefore, it is important to look at what is really required by a practicum site or agency before deciding which form(s) of progress notes will be helpful to the trainee's learning experience.

Lastly, there are limits to what reasonably should be included in art therapy progress notes. Supervisees are being taught to write client progress notes responsibly and sensitively as an art therapist and are not generally expected to conduct and write psychological or psychiatric reports at their practicum or internship site. Diagnostic information is often the responsibility of other professionals on the treatment team, unless the student is being trained specifically for an additional credential upon graduation or through a postgraduate internship (e.g. clinical counseling, marriage & family therapy, or social work) or if the supervisee is required to conduct psychological or developmental assessments as part of his/her internship or job.

Some additional examples of progress note formats are included at the end of this chapter (see figures I & II). Because many psychiatric systems of charting do not account for family work, a guideline for family treatment progress notes developed by Shirley Riley is presented (see Form I). Also, a sample format (see Form II, Process Note Format) for recording therapist-client interactions, the client's reaction to therapy, and the therapist's reaction to the client is included. The reader is also referred to Malchiodi (1990) who has developed a simple format for recording children's responses to art experiences within a non-clinical setting (shelters and facilities for children exposed to family violence). This format can be easily adapted for use with other child populations.

## A Brief Note on Art Expressions & Progress Notes

Regarding art expressions, in some situations the trainee may be required to document art products either by brief description of content or by inclusion or retention of art expressions as part of a client's permanent file. However, most agencies do not seem to consider the retention of client art to be relevant unless the art expression is important to support a diagnosis or to substantiate abuse or trauma. In reality, most facilities cannot physically house, file or store most client artwork due to space, nor do they want to. In contrast, the current AATA ethics document (1995) (see Appendix) considers client art a part of record-keeping, although it is not specific as to what form of record-keeping to which art therapists should adhere (e.g. retain all actual art, retain photos of all art, etc.). Since there are no clear answers for how and what to include in progress notes, supervisors should work with supervisees to develop a realistic plan for record-keeping with regard to art expressions. This plan should satisfy both the facility's needs and the learning experience of the trainee, and above all, respect the client's rights to the art produced.

## Case Studies & Presentations

Case studies and presentations have been a traditional staple of art therapy training, particularly as part of supervisory courses for graduate-level trainees. Often a significant part of the grade for a course involves the completion of a written, lengthy case study and perhaps an accompanying oral presentation to the class. Despite the regular inclusion of such assignments in the training of all therapists, there is very little written to support that case studies are of help in learning to become a therapist (Biggs, 1988). However, educators and supervisors in most helping professions still include case studies within training and completion of at least one client case history continues to be a 'rite of passage' into professionalism.

Case studies are very similar to preparing traditional psychological reports in style and format. The major goal of writing case studies and making oral case presentations is to improve the supervisee's skills in conceptualization of clinical work and the client's process of therapy. If appropriately structured it can also help the trainee develop divergent thinking and problem-solving strategies. According to Biggs (1988), using the case presentation approach deals with three conceptualization tasks: "1) identifying and differentiating how observations and inferences provide evidence for clinical judgments; 2) describing the components of the counseling relationship; and 3) describing a treatment plan including a description of the client's personality, problem condition, factors influencing the problem condition, and choice of intervention strategies" (p.240).

Seasoned educators and supervisors may be a little squeamish about reading (or for that matter, assigning) students' case studies. Having read or listened to literally hundreds of case presentations from both students and professionals, as an educator and supervisor I realize that what bothers me most about case studies are the rambling, extensive narratives which they often contain. Students' case studies are not the only culprits; many of the client histories presented in theses, journals and texts suffer from similar problems. If a case study is to have a purpose, then it must be given a direction and structure in order to provide a meaningful learning experience, as well as keep the reader involved and engaged in the case history of the client. Often just limiting the scope of the study to a set of specifically defined factors helps in this regard.

There is some confusion about the difference between case reporting and actual research which involves the reporting of case materials as part of a larger project. Part of this confusion stems from the use of case studies as final papers or theses for graduate level training. It is important that trainees as well as supervisors understand that case presentations are clinically based observations and not necessarily formal research unless they follow a specific qualitative research paradigm or design.

## Preparing a Case Presentation

Written and oral case presentations have been a tradition in group supervisory sessions, yet very little has been written in the field of art therapy on what constitutes a good case presentation. The purpose of this section is to present an outline for developing an oral and/or written case study and some of the ethical considerations in presenting client material in a classroom or supervisory session.

### Sample Case Presentation Outline

The following outline is offered as a template for components to be included in a formal case study or oral presentation. Supervisors and instructors may wish to add or delete topics to this outline, depending on goals and the trainee's requirements.

## I. AGENCY/FACILITY:

Describe the structure of the agency/facility, including staffing hierarchy.

Describe the services provided by agency.

What referral sources are used by the agency/facility (e.g. how are clients referred into or out of agency/facility)?

Describe the role of student/intern in the agency/facility (e.g. the role of the art therapy trainee within the facility).

## II. POPULATION(S) SERVED BY THE AGENCY/FACILITY:

Description of the student's/intern's case load.

General characteristics (if pertinent): psychological, physical, socio-economic, and any additional demographic information.

## III. CLIENT (subject of the case study):

Describe why you selected this client to discuss through this case study.

Describe the client including the following:

• age

• race (if in doubt of term personally acceptable to the client, ask what is acceptable), e.g. African American/Black, Anglo/Causcasian/White, Asian/Asian-American, Hispanic /Latino, Native American, biracial, etc.

• gender

• religion, if applicable and relevant

• occupation if applicable

• living circumstances, e.g. alone or with family; what kind of setting, e.g. independent housing, halfway house, residential home, etc. Are there caregivers involved?

• if there is a diagnosis, what is it?

• statement of the presenting problem of client; this may include statements from the client describing why treatment is being sought, and the duration, progression and/or severity of problem and assessment of underlying problem

• medical history if applicable (if a more detailed medical history is required, see Zuckerman (1994) for protocols)

•psychiatric history if applicable, including past treatments and professional help sought, hospitalizations

•medications currently taking

•if family work is involved, the construction of a genogram may be included (see McGoldrick & Gerson, 1987, or Zuckerman, 1994, for more information)

•if applicable, a treatment contract made with the client describing the goals and course of action

## IV. SUMMARY OF COURSE OF TREATMENT:

Overall legal and/or ethical considerations in treatment.

Theories/theorists who influenced your treatment plans.

Short and long-term goals as established in the beginning of treatment.

Short and long-term goals as they changed with treatment.

Interventions used to achieve goals.

Whether goals were achieved and how they were achieved.

Termination of treatment, e.g. where is the client going from here?

## V. CONCLUSION:

Overall assessment of this experience.

What did you learn about yourself and yourself as an art therapist because you worked with this client? Because you did this case study?

Other aspects that instructors and supervisors may want trainees to address in a case study include: significant transference and countertransference reactions within the therapeutic relationship (for those operating from psychoanalytic models), sensory, perceptual, spatial abilities, motor skills and cognitive and memory skills. Inclusion of any or all of these aspects will depend on the purpose of the case study, the client population and the goals for the trainee's learning experience.

It is advisable from the outset to provide trainees with the exact format and style of written presentation for completing a case study. Instructors and supervisors may want to refer students to the Publication Manual of the American Psychological Association (1994) or other manuals on the preparation of papers or reports. It is also helpful to give students a short introduction to scholarly writing through a brief list of major requirements (typed, double-spaced, one inch margins, cover sheet); this practice will prevent many problems and misunderstandings later (see Chapter 15 for more information on writing style, including APA style).

## Writing about Clients

In order to accurately write about clients in clear, correct, and concise language, supervisees should be introduced to the available sources of information on clinical terminology. *The American Psychiatric Association Diagnostic and Statistical Manual of Mental Disorders (4th Ed.)* (1994) is a recognized source of clinical terminology. Other resources for writing reports, progress notes and case studies include Zuckerman's (1994) *The Clinician's Thesaurus: A Guidebook for Wording Psychological Reports and Other Evaluations* and *Writing Psychological Reports* by Wolber and Carne (1993). Although these books are not specifically geared to writing about art therapy per se, they do provide standard formats for writing about clients seen in clinical settings such as hospitals or clinics. Because clinical writing is best described in detail by these and other sources, the reader is referred to the list of texts on this subject in the references at the end of this chapter.

In writing about clients in both clinical and non-clinical settings, there are several considerations that should be addressed before assigning case presentations to supervisees. One major issue is the understanding and use of non-biased language in client reports. There are several excellent resources on the use of non-biased language in writing about clients; this material is an important component of learning to prepare a client report which is culturally-sensitive and gender-correct. The American Psychological Association has published several position papers to address the need for sensitivity in how therapists discuss their clients, both culturally (APA, 1991) and with regard to gender (Committee on Lesbian and Gay Concerns, 1991). Supervisors and instructors should consider having these documents on reserve so that students can read them before beginning any writing assignments concerning clients.

Spaniol and Cattaneo (1994) observed the need to raise critical awareness of "how biases become imbedded in language, how language usage maintains differences in power, and how to monitor language use in professional practice" (p. 266). Although these authors focus on the therapeutic relationship, what they have to say is important to how therapists write about clients. For example, they remind us that cultural differences may set up a dynamic in which the non-dominant culture (as defined by race, class, or gender) is defined by the dominant culture (e.g. generally white middle and upper class professionals). They also underscore the importance of sensitivity in talking and writing about mental illnesses, reminding therapists that diagnostic terms are derived from pathology, rather than descriptive of functionality. Spaniol and Cattaneo advocate the use of non-judgmental language; they explain that:

> "Sometimes mental health professionals use language that has negative or fatalistic implications. For example, a term used frequently is the adjective chronic,

which implies that a person can never recover. It is more accurate and less harmful to use such words as prolonged, persistent, serious, or severe because no one can predict the certain course for any individual.... Similarly, when communicating about clients, we can choose to emphasize strengths rather than weaknesses and abilities rather than disabilities, because negative characterizations can become self-fulfilling prophecies." (1994, p. 269)

## Writing About Art Expressions

One aspect that makes writing about art therapy somewhat different from other disciplines is the inclusion of art expressions in most papers and certainly as a major part of most case studies. Often, authors refer to client art in regard to characteristics such as form, style, and content. There is a tremendous need for accuracy in how these art expressions are described.

Both trainees and professionals often rely on the observations made by others about the graphic characteristics of art expressions and sometimes cite this material with reference to the client work to be discussed. Particular care must be taken in using such findings. What can be said about an art expression created by one person may not necessarily be extrapolated to another's work (Malchiodi, 1992). Interpretation has traditionally been a major issue in the discussion of client art expressions and there are a wide variety of opinions on how interpretation should be handled, if at all. On the surface, the standard belief of art therapists appears to be that the client interprets the meaning of his/her art expression. Invariably, however, there often seems to be speculation on the part of both therapists and students as to the meaning of the client's art product. This is not as problematic as it seems if care is taken to differentiate between client observations and statements, and therapist inferences. Many trainees (even some novice supervisors and seasoned professionals) are overzealous in their discussions of art expressions produced by their clients, often stepping into generalizations that cannot be substantiated or, in fact, create unfair and even harmful clinical reports of their clients.

## Oral Presentations of Case Studies

At some point in every student-therapist's education, the trainee has to make one or more case presentations to a class or supervisory group. This ritual is an established part of becoming a therapist in all professions and serves as a place for exploring one's observations within a larger group and receiving feedback from that group. It also is an exercise in learning how to convey information orally, preparing one to communicate client observations to other professionals at internship sites or later, in the workplace or at professional conferences.

Many trainees can experience a great deal of anxiety and even fright about their first oral presentation. Instructors and supervisors should be sensitive to these feelings, remembering what it was like to stand up in front of peers and mentors for the first time to speak about new and complicated materials. Most trainees need a lot of support as well as structure to make initial case presentations a successful learning experience. Giving a clear structure for what is to be presented and how the presentation will be evaluated can alleviate at least some of the fears.

One of the major problems in oral case presentations often involves the issue of time. For example, when the time for presenting a case is limited to 20-30 minutes, the trainees' will often think this amount seems frightfully long, wondering how they will ever fill up the time talking about their client. However, it usually turns out that the student does not plan for the allotted time, leaving the student rushed to come to any concluding remarks in the presentation. Part of this experience comes from the belief that the case that the trainee is presenting is undoubtedly the most interesting case ever known to the field of mental health. But, for the most part, it is a result of poor planning and not practicing the material in advance of presentation. Therefore, it is important to emphasize that the material must be presented in the time allowed and that a couple of practice sessions in front of the mirror or before friends is helpful, too. Since the major reason for giving an oral presentation of this type is to learn how to convey clinical material briefly and concisely to professional peers, it is an important area to emphasize to trainees who will hopefully continue to present later in their career lives, either at conferences or in the workplace.

## Showing Art Expressions as Part of a Case Presentation

Using art expressions as part of case presentations certainly enhance the communication of the trainee's experience with the client to the supervisor and members of a supervision group. In group supervision, art expressions are an excellent way to learn about a variety of client populations and intervention strategies. However, several issues must be carefully taken into consideration when including art expressions as part of oral and/or written case materials.

Permission to share art expressions comes from the client and it is standard to get a signed release form from the client (see Appendix for some sample forms). In the case of minors or those individuals who are unable to grant permission for reason of disability or other condition, parental or guardian permission is required. However, because of the inherent position of power and authority held by the therapist within the therapeutic relationship, careful consideration must be given to the use of art expressions from any client, of any age or status. Spaniol (1994) advocates the use of active and mutual negotiation when obtaining permission from a client to use his/ her art, thus treating the client as a collaborator rather than a research subject or patient to be cured. Through actively negotiating the use of art expressions with the client for specific and/or defined purposes such as case presentations, exhibits, or educational purposes, some of the inherent issues of control, authority, confidentiality, and trust can be addressed through mutual consent and discussion with the client. Because Spaniol's ideas reflect many of the questions about the use and display of client art within the supervisory setting, they are important concepts for supervisors to discuss with all trainees, at all levels. These are issues at the foundation of the art therapy relationship and underscore the importance of the therapist's respect of both clients and their art expressions.

Confidentiality is another topic often at the forefront of ethical discussions concerning client art expressions. Within trainee supervision groups, confidentiality of art expressions (or other client case materials, such as the client's history) among group members is often difficult to maintain. For example, several students may have worked with the same client(s) due to each being assigned the same internship site at different times. In such cases the client's art will be easily recognizable by other trainees and lack of confidentiality cannot be avoided in such cases. However, confidentiality within the group can be maintained and emphasized through use of a confidentiality statement (see Appendix) that each group member signs at the beginning of supervision. This type of written commitment may help to maintain confidentiality concerning material discussed in supervisory settings.

Lastly, the professional display of art expressions is an important component of case presentations. How art expressions are handled, cared for, stored and displayed are part of learning respect for the client's work and the images themselves. Over the years I have seen drawings brought to a class or meeting which have been folded in halves or have dog-eared edges and have been horrified to see the therapist's writing on the client's drawing or painting. A great deal of the self-respect that a client gains from the experience of art therapy is in seeing how respectfully their work is presented and displayed (Malchiodi, 1990). Art may be presented in the form of actual work (e.g. the drawing, painting, etc.), slides or photographs, photocopies (color or black & white) or some sort of facsimile (e.g. hand-drawn sketch approximating the actual art). The way it is presented will depend on whether the client wishes to keep the actual art, and the size and transportability of the piece. However, in all cases the display of the artwork should be done respectfully and with the consideration one would give one's own work.

## Evaluating Case Presentations

Since giving a case presentation is often a significant part of a student's grade for an internship experience, a clear and structured evaluation should be used to assess if the student has met the goals of this learning experience. In most cases, the instructor/supervisor will probably want to give feedback in both verbal and written formats (see end of this chapter for a suggested format). The format for evaluation should be given to the student in advance, along with the assignment. This will make it clear as to exactly what the instructor/supervisor expects and provides trainees with additional information on what to emphasize in their presentations.

If supervision occurs within a group setting, it is often helpful for trainees to give each other feedback in the form of verbal support, questions and challenging discourse, as well as written observations about the presentation (also see the end of this chapter for a suggested peer evaluation format). The supervisor may also want to review the written comments that trainees give each other in order to provide additional feedback on ability to listen, ask appropriate questions, and develop critical thinking skills.

Peer evaluations are also excellent training ground for learning how to supervise others. Supervisees not only benefit from receiving feedback and support from their peers, but also by learning how to give others helpful and proactive direction and suggestions. By learning to give feedback in a supportive, structured, and positive manner, trainees can practice communication skills necessary to be in a supervisory role someday. In using peer evaluation effectively, the supervisor's immediate responsibility is to convey to the trainee's the importance of sensitive, but objective feedback to their peers. If a competitive or insecure environment exists, then the peer evaluation system will obviously not be workable.

## Conclusion

This chapter presents a very brief introduction to clinical writing, documentation, and case presentations. Charting, progress notes, and case histories are usually not the most exciting or inspiring parts of work with clients; however, in clinical settings, both supervisor and supervisee must be knowledgeable and effective in the areas of notation and reporting because of the agency's needs for accurate record-keeping and ethical and legal reasons for maintenance of client files.

Case histories, studies and presentations are usually part of the academic training of the student. However, the skills learned in written and oral presentation of case materials will be useful throughout the therapist's career. Students and seasoned professionals may find themselves providing an inservice workshop to their practicum sites, presenting a case to a treatment team or staff, or giving a paper at a conference or meeting of their peers or related health care professionals. However, the real skill in learning to write progress notes or case materials involves the honing of one's critical thinking skills. By putting thoughts down on paper, within a structure, helps develop new ideas for future treatment, problem-solving and conceptualizing a plan of action on behalf of the clients we serve.

## References:

American Art Therapy Association. (1995). *Ethical standards for art therapists.* Mundelein, IL: Author.

Biggs, D. (1988). The case presentation approach to supervision. *Counselor Education & Supervision, 27,* 240-248.

Malchiodi, C.A. (1990). *Breaking the silence: Art therapy with children from violent homes.* New York: Brunner/ Mazel.

Malchiodi, C.A. (1992). Writing about art therapy for professional publications. *Art Therapy: Journal of the American Art Therapy Association, 9,* (2), 62-64.

McGoldrick, M., & Gerson, R. (1987). *Genograms in family assessment.* New York: Norton.

Spaniol, S. (1994). Confidentiality reexamined: Negotiating use of art by clients. *American Journal of Art Therapy, 32* (3), 69- 74.

Spaniol, S., & Cattaneo, M. (1994). The power of language in the art therapeutic relationship. *Art Therapy: Journal of the American Art Therapy Association, 11*(4), 266-270.

Wolber, G., & Carne, W. (1993). *Writing psychological reports.* Sarasota, FL: Professional Resource Press.

Zuckerman, E. (1995). *Clinician's thesaurus: The guidebook for writing psychological reports.* New York: The Guilford Press.

## Suggested Readings:

American Psychiatric Association. (1994). *Diagnostic and statistical manual of mental disorders* (4th ed.). Washington, DC: Author.

American Psychological Association (1994). *Publication manual of the American Psychological Association* (4th ed.). Washington, DC. Author.

American Psychological Association (1991). *Guidelines for providers of psychological services to ethnic, linguistic, and culturally diverse populations.* Washington, DC. Author. (Developed by the Board of Ethnic Minority

Affairs Task Force on the Delivery of Services to Ethnic Minority Populations)

Committee on Lesbian and Gay Concerns. (1991). Avoiding heterosexual bias in language. *American Psychologist, 46* (9), 973-974.

Deegan, P. (1993). Recovering our sense of value after being labeled. *Journal of Psychiatric Nursing, 31* (4), 7-11.

Research and Training Center on Independent Living. (1993). *Guidelines for reporting and writing about people with disabilities* (3rd. ed.). Lawrence, KS: University of Kansas.

Wolber, G., & Carne, W. (1993). *Writing psychological reports.* Sarasota, FL: Professional Resource Press.

Zuckerman, E. (1995). *Clinician's thesaurus: The guidebook for writing psychological reports.* New York: The Guilford Press.

# Family Treatment Progress Notes

## I. General Information

Provide a brief history of the family

When did the presenting problem become a problematic situation for the family?

Who sees it as a problem?

How did you and the family set goals for treatment?

When you consider your hypothesis for treatment, which theoretical approach appears to fit the family's needs and appear to be syntonic with their version of reality?

Does one person seem to be the symptom-bearer?

Does one person or persons seem to be more anxious to engage the family in treatment than the others?

How do you imagine the family perceives you?

## II. Weekly Progress Notes:

### A. Beginning of the Session

How did the session begin?

What did the clients present to you at the beginning of the conversation?

How did you take advantage of this dialogue by incorporating an art experiential that provided an immediate focus to contain or address the difficulties expressed?

Did this information (e.g. the art product) modify the goals set for treatment?

How do you now assess the family system?

### B. During the Session

What happened during the session?

Describe the interaction between clients, their description of the meaning contained in the art expression, their verbal interactions, etc.

Describe your (silent) interpretation of any second-level meanings revealed or covert implications in the imagery or narratives.

What are the key issues of this family/client?

How many persons agree on the definition of the key issue?

Do you agree with their description(s)?

As the session progressed, did you find opportunities to direct the family/client toward short or long term goals?

Do you feel that you are co-creating the therapeutic outcome with the family/client?

## C. Summary of Session

Describe the family's/ client's summary of the session.

Describe your summary of the session.

Does the theoretical approach you originally selected still seem to address the needs of this family/client?

What gains or failures in treatment would you benefit from discussing in supervision or consultation?

# PROCESS NOTE FORMAT

This format is not for weekly notes per se, but as an exercise in looking more closely at the dynamics, issues and therapist's responses to a 1:1 session with a client. In order to be effective, it requires that the therapist audio or preferably video tape the session in order to record verbatim what was said and how the client and therapist reacted to each other throughout the meeting.

| Participants | Verbal Exchange | Client Behavior | Your Feelings |
|---|---|---|---|
| Therapist | How are you today? | | Slightly anxious. |
| Client | I feel rotten and I don't want to be here today with you. | Looking away from therapist. | More anxious & frustrated. |

# CASE PRESENTATION EVALUATION FORM

## 1. Overall Case Presentation

a) Provides a clear, concise and organized presentation

                                           1    2    3    4    5

b) Includes relevant history (previous treatment, present life circumstances, symptoms, medical data, family, etc.) and presents in a clear format

    1    2    3    4    5

c) Clearly formulates the presenting problem

    1    2    3    4    5

d) Demonstrates an understanding of why the client sought treatment

    1    2    3    4    5

e) Demonstrates understanding of how the client's history relates to the presenting problems    1    2    3    4    5

f) Demonstrates understanding of client's motivation for treatment

    1    2    3    4    5

g) Demonstrates understanding of the client's resistance to treatment

    1    2    3    4    5

h) Demonstrates understanding of the client-therapist relationship and how this may relate to the client's presenting problem, history and interactional style    1    2    3    4    5

i) Provides clear examples from progress notes that relate to the development of the case    1    2    3    4    5

j) Demonstrates understanding of theory as it is applied to therapeutic process

    1    2    3    4    5

Comments:_____

_____

_____

_____

## 2. Treatment Goals

a) Defines both client and therapist treatment goals

    1    2    3    4    5

b) Set short-term, intermediate and long-term goals

    1    2    3    4    5

c) Translate goals in observable and measurable outcomes

    1    2    3    4    5

d) Is able to change goals over the course of treatment as needed

    1    2    3    4    5

Comments:_____
_____
_____
_____

## 3. Execution of Interventions
a) Has clear rationale for providing interventions
                                    1    2    3    4    5

b) Appropriately paces interventions to client's abilities and current status
                                    1    2    3    4    5

c) Chooses interventions with a clear understanding of time restrictions, frequency of sessions, etc.     1    2    3    4    5

d) Chooses interventions with a clear understanding of materials and media variables     1    2    3    4    5

e) Considers alternative interventions
                                    1    2    3    4    5

f) Understands limitations and possible negative consequences of interventions used     1    2    3    4    5

Comments:_____
_____
_____
_____

## 4. Treatment of Art Expressions
a) Obtains appropriate permission for display and presentation
                                  1    2    3    4    5

b) Treats art expressions with care and ethical responsibility
                                  1    2    3    4    5

c) Follows procedures for confidentiality
                                  1    2    3    4    5

d) Discusses art expressions with respect for client and the art expression
                                  1    2    3    4    5

e) Demonstrates understanding of theory with regard to the content of art expressions     1    2    3    4    5

Comments:_____
_____
_____
_____

## 5. Progress Evaluation
a) Has clear criteria for the evaluation of progress

                                                 1    2    3    4    5

b) Checks progress with client

                                                 1    2    3    4    5

c) Check progress with colleagues/supervisors

                                               1    2    3    4    5

d) Revises goals and interventions as necessary

                                               1    2    3    4    5

e) Can support a link between the therapist's interventions and the outcome of treatment        1    2    3    4    5

Comments:_____

_____

_____

_____

## 6. Professionalism
a) Therapist uses good case management skills

                                               1    2    3    4    5

b) Therapist is aware of potential ethical and legal issues relevant to case

                                               1    2    3    4    5

c) Therapist presents case material in ethical and professional manner

                                               1    2    3    4    5

d) Therapist demonstrates ethical and responsible involvement with colleagues and agency        1    2    3    4    5

e) Therapist responds to instructor's questions with appropriateness and professionalism        1    2    3    4    5

Comments:_____

_____

_____

_____

Any additional comments:_____

_____

_____

_____

_____

# PEER EVALUATION FORM/CASE PRESENTATIONS

Name of Student Presenting:_____

Date _____

Please give student feedback in the following areas (5 being highest score):

Delivery of Presentation:
1. Introduced the case study clearly and effectively

           1     2     3     4     5

2. Used clinical terminology appropriately

           1     2     3     4     5

3. Organized case material effectively

           1     2     3     4     5

4. Was able to respond to questions effectively

           1     2     3     4     5

5. Demonstrated critical thinking in discussing the case

           1     2     3     4     5

6. Used client art appropriately and effectively within the presentation

           1     2     3     4     5

Comments about delivery:_____
_____
_____
_____

What professional qualities/abilities do you think that the presenter brings to therapeutic work? (e.g. enthusiasm, creativity, objectivity, etc.)

_____
_____
_____
_____

Please list one recommendation that you have for the presenter regarding this case presentation and any comments you have about this case.

_____
_____
_____

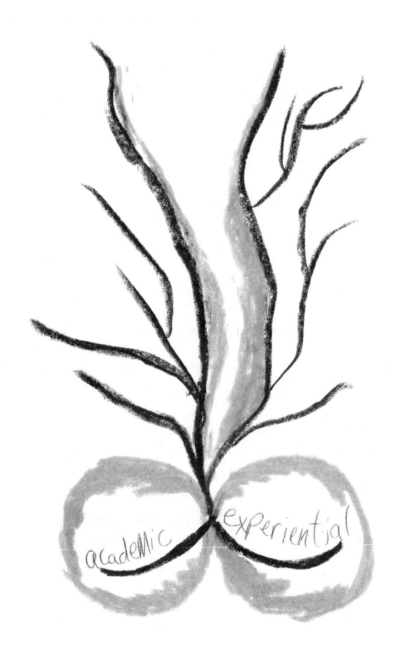

Supervision: Two seeds growing together.

# CHAPTER TWELVE

## Addressing Professional Issues in Art Therapy Training and Supervision
by Cathy A. Malchiodi

The purpose of this chapter is to highlight ways that educators and supervisors can introduce professional issues into the training and/or supervision of art therapy students and supervisees. Professional issues may include, but are not limited to the following topics: credentials and licensure, health care systems and organizations, association 'politics', professional identity and relationships with other clinicians, and trends in clinical practice. Professional issues can also peripherally include ethical dilemmas and legal aspects of practice, although these are areas of study in their own right (and are addressed in other chapters of this book).

On the whole, art therapy graduate students and art therapists in general are poorly versed in professional issues. For example, although art therapy has recently moved into the areas of certification (see various issues of the ATCB Review) and licensure (Good, 1993), most art therapists are naive about both the benefits and the consequences of becoming certified and/or licensed; in fact, many do not even have a basic understanding of the difference between the two or the relative importance of either credential in the health care market. Additionally, art therapists are not usually knowledgeable about health care systems (e.g. for-profit hospitals), health care organizations (e.g. JCAHO), or current trends in mental health service delivery (e.g. managed care, HMOs). These are a few of many areas that educators and supervisors should consider introducing to and discussing with their students through training or supervision sessions.

Advanced art therapy graduate students and postgraduate supervisees are the best candidates for introduction to professional issues. Generally, as a student gets closer to graduation, these issues are of greater interest because the student will soon join the professional ranks and have practical questions about credentials, the job market, and clinical practice. Postgraduate supervisees will also bring concerns about professional issues to supervisory sessions as they mature in their clinical skills, apply for credentials, and begin to interact with others in the field.

## Some Basic Caveats for Supervisors and Educators

A key point for supervisors and educators to remember when introducing professional issues to students is the importance of an open mind in their presentation. We each have, at times, very specific opinions about these topics, due to our own life experiences and training as clinicians. Therefore, it is difficult to present some of these topics without also being somewhat biased in our interpretation. As with any academic material it is important to create responsive formats for exploration and critical thinking about the topics to be considered. Since there are no easy or correct answers for these issues, the student should be provided opportunities to explore them in ways in which personal opinions are freely formulated.

Also, addressing professional issues within the training and/or supervision of students requires that the supervisor or seminar leader stay current in his/her own reading in order to be effective in discussing them. For this reason, some instructors are hesitant to include them in education and training because to gather materials to create such a syllabus takes a great deal of time and a willingness to be knowledgeable about contemporary trends. Since professional issues change so frequently and with time, it is necessary to review the syllabus every so often, adding new readings and topics and discarding that which is outdated.

In the spirit of encouraging educators and supervisors to introduce professional issues in their teaching and supervision, an annotated bibliography is provided at the end of this chapter as a resource. It may be used for the development of a syllabus for a course on professional issues in art therapy or may serve as suggested readings on specific topics for postmasters supervisees.

## Identifying Conceptual Areas for Discussion

After an initial exploration of this subject several years ago I created a semester-long seminar for graduate students on the topic of professional issues in art therapy. Some of the conceptual areas selected for the course syllabus included the following:

- Credentials
- Professional associations (AATA, ACA, AAMFT, ADTA, etc.)
- Identity as an art therapist, relationship to other professionals
- Expanded job settings
- Health care systems/organizations
- Trends in clinical practice

This is certainly not an inclusive list of all possible topics related to professional issues in the field of art therapy. However, given the limited time-frame for study and discussion as well as considering the interests of graduate-level students, it is a good starting place for a beginning dialogue. The rationale for choosing these specific issues follows:

**1. Credentials:** Questions often arise both during graduate supervision and later at the postmasters level about registration, certification, and licensure. Supervisees are often mystified (as are many longtime professionals) about procedures for registration, certification, and licensure, what the differences are, and what the relative importance of each is. With changes in health care and state laws that may restrict the practice of unlicensed therapists, it is important that supervisees be informed about credentials and the various requirements for obtaining them early in their training programs. Also, students and supervisees should have a working knowledge about how credentials relate to competence and what various credentialing processes involve (e.g. training, internship hours, postgraduate work, examination ).

This is not to suggest that the educator/supervisor spend valuable time in a seminar setting helping students/supervisees to fill out forms for registration, for example. What is important, however, is that students understand what the differences in each credential are and are helped to critically think about which credentials are important for him/her. Additionally, in states where there is licensure (whether for art therapy, counseling, marriage and family therapy), a discussion of the particular licensures and professional issues related to licensure is also important; this will obviously vary within training programs and according to state laws. If time permits it is interesting to compare various requirements for professional credentials in related fields (e.g. other creative arts therapists, counselors, etc.) to give students an understanding of the credentials of other clinicians with whom they work.

As a secondary focus, it is important to initiate discussion on the relative importance of professional credentials. There are a great many factors effecting the health care market and it is important that students understand these factors in relation to their own goals for employment. Some examples include: whether certification/licensure is a personal necessity, what credentials are required to be in private practice, and what can be expected to be gained from obtaining specific credentials. Again, the discussion should be an open one, allowing students to explore as much as possible the various reasons for or against obtaining a specific professional credential. An excellent catalyst for such discussion is Corey, Corey, and Callanan (1993) who present arguments both for and against licensing and certification, in addition to some of the other articles mentioned in the bibliography.

**2. Becoming an Active Member of Professional Associations:** An understanding of one's professional association and how to effectively participate as a member of it are important steps in becoming a professional. Some educators/supervisors feel that it is not their place to encourage their students/supervisees to become active in their professional associations. However, considering the rapid changes that are taking place in credentials, licensure, health care systems, governmental affairs, and training, it is extremely important that active participation in association activities be encouraged; the long-term outcome will be more informed and politically involved art therapists.

There is a great deal of 'dry' material available for introducing students to the AATA; specifically, the association bylaws, general membership information, and other documents of general interest. However, what is most important is to convey to students and supervisees how to use their professional association as a source of information and as a network with other art therapists. Additionally, other associations' documents and activities may be important to introduce, particularly if the training program involves dual philosophies (e.g. counseling, marriage and family therapy) or if the state licensure is in a discipline other than art therapy.

**3. Identity and Relationship to Other Professionals:** Discussing, clarifying, and refining one's identity as a therapist is a natural part of a student's maturation into a professional. Since art therapy is still struggling to be a discipline in its own right (Malchiodi, 1993), the question of identity may be harder to answer for art therapists than related health care professionals. Therefore, it is a particularly important area to address in both training and supervision. Some training programs have initiated coursework that satisfies both art therapy registration and licensure requirements in another field, or have advised students to take additional coursework in counseling to meet licensure requirements in that state. There is no doubt that this has compounded questions concerning identity for some students who are less sure of how to simultaneously integrate several disciplines.

Additionally, questions still remain about what role the artist identity plays in art therapy. This has been the subject of debate for many years, with some of the same discussions reemerging from time to time. To a supervisor or advanced professional these discussions may seem repetitive, but remember that supervisees and students are just beginning to face these dilemmas. The struggle with this issue may be at the core of some students' confusion about both theoretical and methodological issues of practice. Often, art therapy literature and debates at national conferences on this issue are not helpful in reducing this anxiety. Therefore, initiating discussion through assigning readings or other activities may help to bring clarity to the struggles many students and novice art therapists experience concerning the integration of art into the therapist's identity.

Lastly, identity issues may also involve the relationship of art therapists to other professionals in health care or other settings (e.g. schools, social services, etc.). It is difficult to work within a setting if one has little understanding of other professionals, administrators, and the general hierarchy. It is also difficult to work within a setting where one's convictions or beliefs are challenged; this is often true for a student or practitioner who is the first art therapist to be employed at a particular facility. Although there are no easy answers, exploration of how an art therapist interfaces with other professionals can help to clarify some of these dilemmas.

**4. Expanded Job Settings:** This is somewhat related to the previous topic of identity, but is more focused on the introduction of new paradigms for service delivery, and new or reinvented roles for art therapists in the job market. Some examples include: alternative health/complementary medicine; businesses and corporations as markets for art therapy; art therapists as artists-in-residence. Readings in this area are harder to find, mostly because much of the material has been presented orally at national conferences. However, *Art Therapy: Journal of the American Art Therapy Association* (see V. 11, #1, 2, 3, &4, 1994) published viewpoints by art therapy 'pioneers' on the future of the profession, some of which discussed how art therapists might be employed in the coming decades.

**5. Health Care:** Health care has been a topic of public scrutiny for the last several years and will probably continue to be throughout the 90's. With the rise of for-profit hospitals and the decline in insurance payment dollars, health care has seen many changes over the last two decades in both service delivery and availability. Important areas for discussion are topics such as managed care, health maintenance organizations, and new changes in health care. A working knowledge of the Joint Commission for Accreditation of Healthcare Organizations (JCAHO), the Accreditation Manual for Hospitals (AMH), and the Consolidated Standards Manual (CSM) is important for art therapy students and postgraduate supervisees (as well as art therapists) who work in hospitals; the Continuous Quality Improvement Manual (Howie & Gutierrez, 1994) is a source of information on these documents.

**6. Trends in Clinical Practice:** The readings in this area are more theoretical, provocative, and philosophical, but worth looking into for discussion purposes. Because this is complex material, they also may be more appropriate to postmaster supervisees rather than art therapy graduate students who usually have more basic concerns. Trends in clinical practice may include material on the future of health care, impact of society on the individual, and multicultural and gender issues. Sources for readings may include editorials, commentaries, and personal viewpoints. Several books listed in the bibliography contain materials related to this theme.

Any or all of these topics can theoretically be included in a class syllabus, combined with assigned readings, experiential work and theme paper(s) on a specific area of study. For postmasters supervisees, these topics may serve as a reference list of possible areas for discussion, recommended reading, or further exploration outside the supervisory session.

Additional sources of articles include association newsletters (American Art Therapy Association, American Counseling Association, American Psychological Association, and American Association of Marriage & Family Therapists, to name a few) and journals (particularly those in the field as well as publications such as the Family Therapy Networker), which focus on contemporary and cutting edge issues in the practice of therapy. Editorials, points of view, commentaries or personal opinions, and committee reports are good places to start a search for material, mainly because their content is often on current developments, debates, or positions.

## Conclusion

Bringing professional issues related to the practice of art therapy into the classroom or supervisory session can be a stimulating addition to training and internship experiences. For students and supervisees, it can enhance not only their overall understanding of their profession and their colleagues, but also the health care systems, complex regulations, and changing trends in service delivery. For instructors/supervisors, introducing professional issues into the supervision or training of art therapy students/supervisees can be a challenging task. It is one requiring an open mind and a dedication to staying current in not only the field of art therapy, but also in health care, changing regulations, and events that impact the provision of therapy in general. This is a difficult and time-consuming task, but is one that will benefit the student or supervisee as well as the entire field by training therapists to be critical thinkers and contemporary in their understanding of clinical practice.

## References

Corey, G., Corey, M., & Callanan, P. (1993). *Issues and ethics in the helping professions.* Pacific Grove, CA: Brooks/Cole.

Good, D. (1993). The history of art therapy licensure in New Mexico. *Art Therapy: Journal of the American Art Therapy Association, 10*(3), 136-140.

Malchiodi, C.A. (1993). Is there a crisis in art therapy education? *Art Therapy: Journal of the American Art Therapy Association, 10* (3), 122-128.

## Annotated Bibliography on Professional Issues

### Professional Credentials:

Alberding, B., Lauver, P., & Patnoe, J. (1993). Counselor awareness of the consequences of certification and licensure. *Journal of Counseling & Development, 72 (1)*, 33-38.

The authors examined the extent to which counselors are familiar with the potential consequences of certification and licensure on their practice. Although counselors are licensed in a majority of states, most surveyed were found to be unfamiliar with the negative aspects of regulation. Given art therapy's increasing involvement in certification and licensure, this is a relevant article for students and supervisees.

Art Therapy Credentials Board (ATCB). (1996). *A.T.R. registration application.* Chicago, IL: Author.

For most supervisors and educators this is a good document to have on hand; however, it is advisable to contact the ATCB once year for an updated copy, since credential requirements may change periodically.

Art Therapy Credentials Board (1996). *Bulletin of information.*Chicago, IL: Author.

This document outlines requirements and procedures for applying for board certification in art therapy. General information, application forms and sample questions are included. It is advisable to contact the ATCB once a year for updated copies.

Art Therapy Credentials Board. (1996). *Certification examination study guide.* Chicago, IL: Author.

Provides additional information on conceptual areas potentially covered in the art therapy certification examination.

Baker, B. (1994, July/August). Art therapy's growing pains. *Common Boundary*, 42-48.

This article brought art therapy's move to create a national certification program into the public and is worth reading as an introduction to the pro's and con's of certification for art therapists.

Corey, G., Corey, M., & Callanan, P. (1993). *Issues and ethics in the helping professions.* Pacific Grove, CA: Brooks/Cole.

See Chapter 7 [Professional Competence & Training], specifically the section on "Professional Licensing and Credentialing" for a very even-handed discussion of the pro's and con's of certification and licensure in the helping professions.

Good, D. (1993). The history of art therapy licensure in New Mexico. *Art Therapy: Journal of the American Art Therapy Association, 10*(3), 136-140.

This article discusses the events that led to the establishment of the first art therapy licensure, explaining the process of writing legislation, introducing a bill to the legislature, and factors pertinent to passage. Personal reflections on the process are included to familiarize readers with how a bill becomes law.

Knapp, J., Knapp, L., & Phillips, J. (1994). Report on the national art therapy practice analysis survey. *Art Therapy: Journal of the American Art Therapy Association, 11*(2), 146-150.

Provides the statistical analysis of the practice survey sent out to all A.T.R.'s in 1993; data derived from this study was used to construct the first certification examination for art therapists.

Malchiodi, C.A. (1994). Sorting out certification. *Art Therapy: Journal of the American Art Therapy Association, 11*(2), 82-83.

Examines the pro's and con's of the development and implementation of a certification examination for art therapists.

New Mexico Counseling and Therapy Board. (1993). *Counselor and therapist practice act.* Santa Fe, NM: Author.

The actual bill passed in 1993 that licensed art therapists by their own title; since this is a governmental document, it is a bit long in the tooth, but informative as both an historical and practical piece on what art therapists can expect from licensure. Because there is no residency clause (as of 1994) art therapists from any state can apply for this credential and for this reason, may want to familiarize themselves with it.

Weinrach, S., & Thomas, K.R. (1993). The National Board for Certifying Counselors (NBCC): The good, the bad and the ugly. *Journal of Counseling & Development, 72* (1), 105-109.

This article outlines the outcomes of the implementation of a national certification for counselors and what has resulted from that decision. It is not entirely complimentary of the counselor certification efforts, but provides interesting perspectives on the relative value of certification in the health care market place.

## Professional Associations:

American Art Therapy Association. (1987). *Model job description*. Mundelein, IL: Author. [This document can also be found in M.B. Junge with P. P. Asawa (1994), A History of Art Therapy in the United States, Mundelein, IL: AATA, Inc.]

American Art Therapy Association. (1992). *Bylaws*. Mundelein, IL: Author. Not exactly exciting reading, but supervisors and educators may want to familiarize students with it and the basic tenets of the AATA's board and committee structure. This document is updated periodically, so be sure to locate the most recent version. [Also available from the AATA National Office: General Membership Information, Resource Sheet, Code of Ethics, Standards of Practice for Art Therapists, Survey Report, and Education and Training Requirements; write to American Art Therapy Association, Inc., 1202 Allanson Road, Mundelein, IL 60060.]

## Addresses for other professional associations (these addresses are subject to change):

American Association for Music Therapy, PO Box 80012, Valley Forge, PA 19484; 610-265-4006

American Dance Therapy Association, 2000 Century Plaza, Suite 108, Columbia, MD 21044; 410-997-4040.

American Society of Group Psychotherapy & Psychodrama. 6728 Old McLean Village, McLean, VA 22101; 703-556-9222.

American Association for Marriage & Family Therapy, 1133 15th Street NW, Washington, DC 20005-2710; 202-452-0109.

American Counseling Association, 5999 Stevenson Avenue, Alexandria, VA 22304; 703-823-9800.

American Psychological Association, 750 First Street NE, Washington, DC 20002; 202-336-5500.

National Art Education Association, 1916 Association Drive, Reston, VA 22091; 703-860-8000.

National Association for Drama Therapy, 2022 Cutter Drive, League City, TX 77573; 713-334-4421.

National Association for Poetry Therapy, PO Box 551, Port Washington, NY 11050.

National Coalition of Arts Therapies Associations, c/o ADTA, 2000 Century Plaza, Suite 108. Columbia, MD 21044; 410-997-4048.

## Professional Identity

Allen, P.B. (1992). Artist-in-residence: An alternative to "clinification" for art therapists. *Art Therapy: Journal of the American Art Therapy Association, 9*(1), 22-29.

Provocative piece on the idea that as art therapists cease to make art, clinical skills gradually become a career focus. The author also offers suggestions to combat "clinification" of art therapists, including a studio approach to art therapy.

Ault, R. (1977). Are you an artist or therapist—A professional dilemma of art therapists. In R. Shoemaker & S. Gonick-Barris (eds.), *Creativity and the Art Therapist's Identity* (pp. 53- 56), Proceedings of the 7th Annual AATA Conference. Baltimore, MD: AATA.

This is an older piece, but outlines a dilemma that continues within the profession. Ault's recounting of his own self-examination of his role as a professional is authentic and will serve as the catalyst for enlivening discussions on this issues in the years to come.

Irwin, E.C. (1986). On being and becoming a therapist. *The Arts in Psychotherapy, 13,* 191-195.

This is a thoughtful, personal piece which addresses how one becomes a good therapist and what it is that therapists do that helps others to feel better and function more effectively.

Johnson, D. (1985). Envisioning the link among the creative arts therapies. *The Arts In Psychotherapy, 12,* 233-238.

Outlines how the creative arts therapies are linked theoretically and methodologically, as well as how political connections between them could strengthen their cumulative position in the health care market.

Junge, M., Alvarez, J. F., Kellogg, A., & Volker, C. (1993). The art therapist as social activist. *Art Therapy: Journal of the American Art Therapy Association, 10*(3), 148-155.

This joint effort by four art therapists explores the idea of the art therapist as an agent of social change. Viewpoints from two art therapists who worked with Central American refugees and one who worked as trade union activist are shared.

Lachman-Chapin, M. (1993). The art therapist as exhibiting artist. *Art Therapy: Journal of the American Art Therapy Association, 10*(3), 141-147.

The author asks the question: Are the identities of artists and art therapists fundamentally opposite? Also cited are the writings of Gablik and Kuspit to support the author's premise.

Malchiodi, C.A., Allen, P.B., & Cattaneo, M. (1991). *Art therapy: Post-mortem.* Opening session presentation at the Annual AATA Conference, Denver, CO. National Audio Video #1-135 [ 4465 Washington Avenue, Denver, CO 80216].

Three art therapists eulogized the profession of art therapy, critically examining professional identity as a whole and presenting a pessimistic view of its future.

Riley, S. (1994). Art therapy in the 21st century. *Art Therapy: Journal of the American Art Therapy Association, 11*(2), 100-101.

A thoughtful piece on the future of art therapy focusing on identity and the possibilities for new identities as art therapists in the coming years.

Sandel, S. (1989). On being a female creative arts therapist. *The Arts in Psychotherapy, 16*, 239-242.

The author explores the gender issues intrinsic to working as a female arts therapist: equal pay, sexual harassment, and the impact of motherhood.

## Expanded Work Settings

Lippin, R.A. (1985). Arts medicine. *The Arts in Psychotherapy, 12*, 147-49.

The author describes the emerging field of arts medicine. Although the description falls heavily on the side of medicine and physicians rather than arts therapies, it is still a paradigm worth considering and exploring within the concept of expanded work settings.

Malchiodi, C.A. (1993). Medical art therapy: Defining the field. *International Journal of Arts Medicine, 2*(1), 28-31.

Offers a definition for medical art therapy based on health psychology, alternative/complementary medicine, and new paradigms in health care.

Smart, M. (1986). Expanded work settings. *Art Therapy: Journal of the American Art Therapy Association, 3*, 21-26.

Challenges art therapists to broaden their definitions of what they do in the workplace and describes the author's experiences with Employee Assistance Programs (EAP) as a potential employment resource.

## Health Care

Freeny, M. (1994). Getting well in the fast lane. *Family Therapy Networker, 18*(2), 73-76.

Futuristic piece that fantasizes mental health service delivery at the turn of the century.

Howie, P., & Gutierrez, K.G. (1994). *The continuous quality improvement manual.* Mundelein, IL: AATA, Inc.

An AATA publication that presents the nuts and bolts of continuous quality improvement (CQI) in hospital settings. A good introduction to JCAHO and other health organizations.

Lipchik, E. (1994). The rush to be brief. *Family Therapy Networker, 18* (2), 34-39.

Trends in brief therapy and its implications for mental health service delivery are explored.

O'Hara, M., & Anderson, W.T. (1991, September/October). Welcome to the postmodern world. *Family Therapy Networker*, 19-25.

An overview of postmodernism and its effect on therapists' practice.

## Trends in Clinical Practice

Gergen, K. (1991). *The saturated self.* New York: Basic Books.

This a provocative book about the postmodern world and the psychological issues that impact self-identity in the 90's. Interesting reading for art therapists both because of the psychological and societal and the infusion of visual art throughout the text.

Hillman, J., & Ventura, M. (1993). *We've had a hundred years of psychotherapy— and the world's getting worse.* San Francisco: Harper San Francisco.

In this popular book, the authors take to task some of the foundations of modern psychotherapy and question the effectiveness of therapeutic intervention in ameliorating both individual and societal problems.

Lerner, M. (1995). The assault on psychotherapy. *Family Therapy Networker, 19* (5), 44-52.

This article on the future of practice poses the question -how did health care turn into health business? and examines the demands of doing therapy within a managed care environment.

Malchiodi, C.A. (1994). Family art therapy and postmodern society. In Riley, S. & C. Malchiodi, *Integrative Approaches to Family Art Therapy* (pp. 213-221). Chicago: Magnolia Street Publishers.

An introduction to the concept of postmodernism as it relates to art therapists and its implication for practice with families in the 90's.

Riley, S. (1994). Change: The reality of the mental health providers' world in the 1990's. In Riley, S. & C. Malchiodi, *Integrative Approaches to Family Art Therapy* (pp. 247-256). Chicago: Magnolia Street Publishers.

This chapter emphasizes the importance of being alert to changes in society and the environment that affect mental health service delivery. Three areas are addressed: training students in legal matters and personal safety, new paradigms for intervention, and involvement in professional associations.

Wadeson, H. (1994). Question: Will art therapy survive universal health coverage reform? *Art Therapy: Journal of the American Art Therapy Association, 11* (1), 26-28.

Although universal health care reform was not implemented in 1994, the author presents many observations about the future of art therapy in a changing health care climate that are well-worth discussion. Among the topics raised are: managed care, private practice, and future employment opportunities for art therapists.

Wylie, M.S. (1994). Endangered species. *Family Therapy Networker, 18* (2), 20-33.

Asks a controversial question: Are psychotherapists becoming an endangered species? This article may make educators uncomfortable as it brings into light the idea that job security in mental health is waning and that salaries are threatened. However, in the interest of giving students and supervisees a real glimpse at what they face, it is a worthwhile addition to a syllabus and may generate lively discussions.

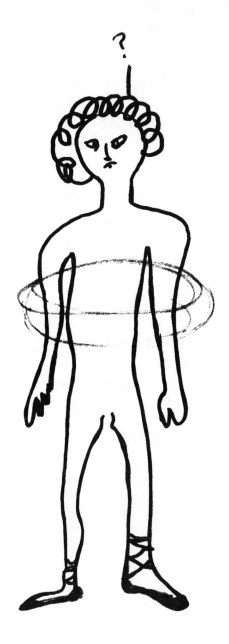

In a bind... not knowing what to do.

# CHAPTER THIRTEEN

## Addressing Ethical and Legal Issues in Art Therapy Training and Supervision
by Cathy A. Malchiodi

The purpose of this chapter is to suggest resources and strategies which educators and supervisors can use to introduce ethical standards and legal issues in training and/or supervision. Both ethics and law are included in this chapter because they are difficult subjects to separate; for example, ethical standards in art therapy and other helping professions are regulated by laws as well as professional codes. However, it has also been observed that ethics involve ideal standards set by professionals, while laws are the minimum standards that society finds acceptable (Corey, Corey & Callanan, 1993).

Since ethical behavior and knowledge of the law are important to every therapeutic interaction, both topics should be introduced to trainees as early as possible in their academic programs, at the very least before students begin an internship or practicum. However, the study of ethics and legal issues can also be extremely overwhelming, given the complexities of both areas and the ever-changing regulations that may affect clinical practice. For first year students who are grappling with the foundations of art therapy as a discipline, certain ethical and legal issues may be hard to comprehend, given the priorities for learning basic theoretical material and skills. Also, most students lack practical experience as clinicians, experience which demonstrates the importance of ethical standards and legal matters as related to work with clients, agencies, and other professionals.

In contrast to student practitioners, postgraduate supervisees more regularly bring both ethical and legal questions to sessions, often dilemmas that involve clients, agencies, and other professionals. Concerns about dual relationships, reporting, duty-to-warn, and personal liability naturally come with the territory of being on one's own as a working professional in health services. It becomes particularly important for supervisors to be responsive to postgraduate supervisees' questions and to be knowledgeable about ethics and the law. A supervisor, by legal definition, is primarily responsible for his/her trainees actions with clients (please see Chapter 14 for a more specific discussion of legal responsibilities of supervisors) .

Although many areas of ethics and regulations can be addressed with supervisees, the following topics are a few of those which are the most common. This list was originally generated for a graduate-level seminar on ethics, but the topics are also appropriate for both advanced graduate students and postgraduate trainees, particularly those trainees who are planning to take either examinations for board certification and/or licensure. Throughout this chapter the reader is referred to materials that may be helpful in generating discussions and answering some of the questions that trainees may have. Following the conclusion, an annotated bibliography on ethics and legal matters is included for this purpose.

Lastly, it is particularly important in the training and supervision of art therapists (as well as those professionals who use art expression as part of therapy) to emphasize the unique ethical and legal aspects that affect art therapy services. As art therapists we differ from other professionals in that we have ethical considerations that involve art expressions and the handling of client art; related health professionals who use art expressions or art making in therapy should also take into consideration these unique ethical considerations. The legal aspects of retention and disposition of client art are complex (see Braverman, 1995; Malchiodi, 1995; Spaniol, 1994), given that art expressions created in therapy can be viewed both as personal expressions at one end of the continuum and as medical records on the other. These are not questions that are easily answered, since the mix of therapy and art making is an unusual blend of treatment and personal expression. However, these obviously are important topics not only in the training and supervision of students, but also in the ongoing clinical work of seasoned practitioners.

## I. Ethics

The American Art Therapy Association has established and regularly updates a document outlining the ethical code for art therapists (see Appendix). It is important to preface this section by stating that ethical codes do not present definite answers to the ethical dilemmas that practitioners face in the course of their work, nor do they communicate the absolute truth. However, they do constitute the available parameters for discussing and learning about ethical behavior and its relationship to client welfare. The following topics are some that are common in supervisory discussions with trainees and professionals:

## Confidentiality

Confidentiality is the "ethical and legal responsibility to safeguard clients from unauthorized disclosure of information given in the therapeutic relationship" (Corey, Corey & Callanan, 1993, p.102 ). Although confidentiality is also a legal issue, it is first an ethical one that is the basis of all therapeutic relationships. It is fair to say that all helping professions have established ethical codes that address confidentiality and privacy. The Ethical Standards for Art Therapists (AATA, 1995 ) is not an exception and states in the section introduction:

> Art therapists shall respect and protect confidential information obtained from patients in conversation and/or through artistic expression.

In most areas, the AATA ethical code is similar to those of other related disciplines: that treatment of clients must be in a private and confidential setting; that disclosure of confidential information without consent is only in matters of danger to the self or others; that disclosure of confidential information is required when mandated by law and only as reasonably necessary.

However, the use of art expression within the therapeutic framework does present some unique situations with regard to confidentiality. For example, Wilson (1987) notes that although therapists can alter biographical information and names to disguise client identities, the uniqueness of art expressions cannot be easily changed to protect a client's privacy. The situation becomes complicated when client art is exhibited with permission in a public place where family or friends may recognize the work, even when the artist's name is removed. Other problems such as making a gift of the art expression to the therapist, or abandoning work when therapy has terminated (Moon, 1994) leaves ethical problems for the art therapist that other clinicians are less likely to face.

Possibly one of the most confusing and controversial aspects of confidentiality in the practice of art therapy has been the maintenance and disposition of client art expressions, concerning which the document states:

> Art therapists shall maintain patient treatment records for a reasonable amount of time consistent with state regulations and sound clinical practice, but not less

than seven years from completion of treatment or termination of the therapeutic relationship. Records are stored or disposed of in ways that maintain confidentiality. (AATA, 1995)

It is difficult to say from reading this statement whether art expressions are considered "treatment records" per se, or if they are, that they must be retained for the stipulated seven year period. In a report to the AATA membership, Braverman (1995) notes that "while it appears that the majority of therapists agree that the patient, indeed, owns the artwork, it is nevertheless true that in many instances artwork may constitute a medical record" (p. 15). When and if art expressions become medical records is an ongoing concern for art therapists, and until it is decided from a legal standpoint, the ethical aspects of retention of client work are important to all art therapists and those who use art expression in therapy. Discussions of retention, storage, and disposition of client art along with the perceptions of clients themselves concerning their art should be continuous topics within supervisory sessions on ethics (Malchiodi, 1995).

Lastly, exhibiting client art is another ethical dilemma faced by art therapists. Even when an agreement and appropriate permissions are received to exhibit work, there are additional ethical considerations to be made. An excellent resource in this area is the work of Spaniol (1990a; 1990b); supervisors and instructors may want to use this author's work in generating discussions concerning public display of client work.

## Using Art Expressions for Assessment Purposes

In 1990, the AATA Board of Directors adopted the following statement concerning art-based assessments:

> Art therapists use a variety of art-based assessments which include, but are not limited to, free choice and/or directed drawings, paintings, and/or sculptures. The choice of the specific art therapy assessment depends on the age of the client and the purpose for which the assessment will be used. Art therapists are aware of the most recent research on assessment and evaluation and of state laws and agency policies which govern the use of assessment procedures. (AATA, 1990)

The area of art-based assessment is both a confusing and complicated issue for trainees as well as professionals. When using art expressions for evaluative purposes, art therapists must be fully cognizant of the seriousness of what they are doing. Some of the projective testing materials that art therapists often base evaluations on are at best archaic (Malchiodi, 1992; 1994). This is irresponsible on the part of both instructors and supervisors who may offer such material to their trainees, as well as any therapist who uses it without first understanding its limitations. Some of the more recent drawing tasks and protocols that are purported to be useful in assessment have not been standardized and have not been fully researched (Malchiodi, 1994).

Given that many art therapists and other health professionals use art expressions to not only understand their clients, but also for assessment, evaluative, and sometimes diagnostic purposes, it is extremely important that they also have a complete understanding of the ethics involved in using these in such a way. For some art therapists the very question of using art expressions for assessment or diagnosis is an ethical one and is a philosophical discussion in and of itself. Also, given the minimal amount of research data available on the exact meaning of art expressions in general, it is still difficult to make a prediction from graphic data without additional information such as client statements or behaviors. Therefore, any use of art expression to assess or evaluate an individual requires therapists be current in their knowledge of research data as well as sensitive to the use of art products to interpret the individual client.

Ethics involved in the interpretation of client art expressions should be included in student training and may be revisited throughout one's postgraduate years as a professional. These include the boundaries of interpretation and respect for the art product (McNiff, 1991), and multicultural issues of interpretation (Cattaneo, 1994), among others. How a client views art expression as opposed to how a therapist sees art expression is also important; clients, especially children, may not necessarily understand that an art assignment may also be a assessment tool (Malchiodi, 1992; 1994). Most client's experiences with art making have been in an educational setting, where the purpose of art expression is often somewhat different than in the average art therapy setting. The idea that art can be used for assessment is familiar to art therapists, but not necessarily to all of their clients, even after informed consent or explanation. Although this type of discussion may be more theoretical and philosophical and not very cut-and-dry, these are issues directly related to the foundations of ethical treatment of art expressions and client welfare.

Although this section specifically deals with the ethics of using art in assessment, there are also legal issues that may be involved. State laws and even agency policies may greatly limit the use of so-called standard projective drawing tasks. There have been scattered reports over the years of art therapists who have been restricted from performing these tasks and using the word "diagnosis" in a description of what they do. Some states have laws that allow the use of assessments and tests by specifically licensed professionals (e.g. psychologists, social workers, counselors). Although many art therapists are trained at the graduate level to perform art-based assessments, laws may prevent their doing so, particularly if they are not licensed. With these thoughts in mind it may be wise to check with state psychological associations and any licensure regulations to see if the use of projectives is limited to use by certain professionals or if art therapists are restricted from using them in any way.

## Dual Relationships

The topic of dual or multiple relationships is one of the most prominent areas of ethical concern across all health professions. Carrigan (1993) notes that an increasing number of formal complaints have been filed to ethical practice boards across all health professions concerning dual or multiple relationships with both trainees and clients. In response to the numerous problems reported in the area of dual relationships, professional associations have included specific guidelines for multiple roles in their ethics codes with reference to training and supervision and work with clients. For example, the American Art Therapy Association states:

> Art therapists shall recognize their influential position with respect to patients, and they shall not exploit the trust and dependency of such persons. A dual relationship occurs when a therapist and patient engage in separate and distinct relationship(s) or when an instructor or supervisor acts as a therapist to a student... (AATA, 1995)

The American Counseling Association (ACA) (1995) also acknowledges that dual relationships should be avoided, but also recognizes that they are difficult to avoid in some circumstances:

> Professional counselors are aware of their influential position with respect to clients, and they avoid exploiting the trust and dependency of clients.... When a dual relationship cannot be avoided, professional counselors take appropriate professional precautions (such as informed consent, consultation, supervision, and documentation) to ensure that judgment is not impaired and no exploitation occurs.

The American Psychological Association expresses similar opinions regarding multiple roles:

> 1.17 Multiple Relationships (APA Code of Ethics, 1993)
>
> a) In many communities and situations, it may not be feasible or reasonable for psychologists to avoid social or other nonprofessional contacts with persons such as patients, clients, students, or supervisees. Psychologists must always be sensitive to the potential harmful effects of other contacts on their work and on those persons with whom they deal. A psychologist refrains from entering into or providing another personal, scientific, professional, financial, or other relationship with such persons if it appears likely that such a relationship reasonably might impair the psychologist's objectivity or otherwise interfere with the psychologist's

effectively performing his or her functions as a psychologist, or might harm or exploit the other party.

Other ethical principles related to multiple roles include not engaging in any type of sexual intimacies with former clients, and refraining from teaching and supervising former clients until a specific amount of time has passed. These are important, but somewhat confusing, rules and should be discussed at length with students and supervisees because of their complexity. To add to the confusion, many codes of ethics differ on various principles, such as the length of time which must pass until a professional may actually serve as a supervisor to a former client. Currently, the AATA document states two (2) years; other documents, state laws, and regulations may stipulate longer time limits.

Because of the multidimensional aspects of dual relationships and the variety of ways ethical codes have addressed this topic, many agencies and academic programs have developed position statements concerning dual relationships to supplement ethical codes. The following guidelines concerning multiple roles were developed by Cattaneo and Gawalek (1994) for faculty and supervisors in a graduate level training program for counseling psychology and expressive therapies. They noted that: 1) teachers and supervisors must recognize the power inherent in the role of teacher and supervisor in situations related to teaching, supervising, and therapy; 2) faculty and supervisors should not engage in any business or social relationships that compromise the student-teacher relationship; 3) faculty and supervisors are responsible for clarifying that clinical training is not psychotherapy; 4) faculty and supervisors will refrain from providing private/independent supervision or therapy to any student currently enrolled in one of their courses or supervision groups; and 5) no faculty member should solicit or advertise clinical services in the classroom setting (e.g. flyers or notices regarding therapy, supervision or training seminars).

Although most ethical codes recommend avoiding dual relationships altogether, it is also recognized that it is difficult to keep counseling out of supervision and clinical training; in fact some see this as practically impossible, given the nature of the dynamic (Ryder & Hepworth, 1990). Wilson (in Wilson, Riley, & Wadeson, 1984) notes that there is a distinction between self-exploration through art making and the self-examination that comes from personal therapy. She emphasizes that the prime directive of supervision is to help the trainee understand how personal problems may interfere with clinical work with clients; it is not, however, to take on the role of therapist with the supervisee. In conveying this concept, most of the vagueness in boundaries between teaching, supervision and therapy can be eliminated. Calisch (1989) takes a slightly different view, stating that "...the supervisor must communicate that attention to interpersonal issues is not only permissible, but is a very important component of the supervisory relationship" (p. 41). She sees interpersonal issues as unavoidable in the supervisor/supervisee relationship and that taking such a stance is a collaborative move which encourages openness between trainer and trainee.

Lastly, with regard to multiple roles in general, it is wise to discuss with trainees some of the most common and potentially problematic dual relationship roles such as bartering for goods and/or services between therapist and client, social relationships with clients or trainees, training friends or relatives, and accepting gifts from clients or trainees. Although these issues are clearly delineated in many ethical codes, there is considerable ambivalence among professionals about following standards as set forth by their professional associations. For example, educators in small departments may wear more than one hat (e.g. supervise, advise, teach, and administrate), making dual relationships with trainees almost impossible to avoid. Therapists who live in small communities, particularly rural areas, also cannot avoid the overlap between professional and personal relationships. Additionally, in some parts of the country, bartering is a common form of payment for services. These are only a few of the many examples where roles may overlap and ethics as well as other factors must be examined. Although these overlapping role relationships are unavoidable, a thorough discussion of the inherent ethical responsibilities is a necessity in all aspects of training and supervision.

## Research & Involvement of Human Subjects

Research issues are more fully discussed in many texts, including the AATA research guide (Wadeson, 1992). Needless to say, ethical standards for conducting research and regard for research participants are important topics within both the training and supervision of art therapists and are already addressed in more detail in other books.

## Standards of Practice

Two documents related to ethics that every supervisor and every supervisee should be familiar with are the General Standards of Practice (AATA, 1989) and the Definition of Independent Practitioner (AATA, 1995). Both documents provide guidelines for art therapists regarding art therapy services and the therapist's relationship to the client, peer professionals, and the larger community. A full discussion of these documents is warranted with graduate-level students; supervisors of postgraduate students will want to revisit them from time to time with their trainees. The latest versions of both documents are included in the Appendix.

## II. Legal Areas

Although there are a variety of laws which affect and regulate health professions, many art therapists are not particularly well-versed in them and what they mean to professional practice. The following are some of the most common areas of law that supervisors and instructors should discuss with trainees:

### Laws Affecting Therapeutic Practice

Laws in some states put specific restrictions on what you can and cannot do as an unlicensed art therapist. Webster (1994), for example, relates her experiences as an unlicensed art therapist in the state of California. She notes that art therapists not licensable under existing categories in that state must be careful about the services that they say they provide. For example, "in the opening orientation [to art therapy] and/or in the informed consent statements given to new clients, care must be taken to state that the unlicensed art therapist who is not supervised is not doing psychotherapy" (p. 280). Other states may have what are referred to as omnibus bills for mental health therapists which may limit who can provide mental health therapy or psychotherapy, and under certain conditions.

Other laws that may affect art therapists, licensed or not, may include rules about advertising and representing oneself to the public, disclosure, privacy and privileged communications, and liability. Although some of these issues are addressed in the Ethical Standards for Art Therapists and other ethical codes, it is still necessary to have a full understanding of state laws which conflict with these documents. Therefore, supervisors, instructors, and trainees must be responsible for knowing what laws exist in their own states that affect therapeutic practice.

### Child Abuse/Neglect and Domestic Violence

Laws that affect the reporting of abuse or violent behavior are an extremely important foundation for trainees. There are laws in each state that govern when and how therapists must report suspected child abuse and domestic violence. As a general rule, all human service professionals are required to report known or suspected child abuse and neglect. Kalichman (1993) also cites that the three greatest difficulties in obeying reporting laws involve who is required to report, what must be reported, and when one must report. Although all state laws are different, mandatory reporting laws across states do have several things in common; the "laws define abusive situations; delineate reportable circumstances, the level of certainty reporters must reach, the age limits of reportable children, and details of who must report; outline sanctions for not reporting; and provide immunity from civil and criminal liability for reports filed in good faith" (Kalichman, 1993, p. 13; also see Meriwether, 1986).

Art therapists may hear children describe actual incidents of abuse to them; it is often likely that they will also see evidence to suspect abuse in the art expressions of children at risk, whether in schools, clinics, or shelter programs (Malchiodi, 1991). Children, especially those who have been chronically abused, may relate this information in a less-than-obvious fashion, either through metaphoric themes in post-traumatic play or drawings that are symbolic of various types of abuse or neglect (Malchiodi, 1990). Although an art therapist may feel an art expression or series of art expressions contains enough information to reasonably suspect that abuse has occurred, it is often difficult to substantiate based on the current dearth of hard data available on children's art products.

Protective services may require verbal verification in addition to behavioral indicators in order to pursue a reported case and may not find art expressions, on their own, acceptable substantiation of abuse/neglect. For those who work in agencies where child abuse reporting is a regular occurrence, several strategies can reduce the level of personal frustration in the referral of such information. First, it is extremely important to make a connection with someone in protective services who you can call upon to assist you in making your report; subsequent reporting will go much more smoothly if you can establish this contact. Second, follow-up on reporting is also important; with the high number of existing caseloads, reports and referrals do become lost or go unaddressed. By assertively (not necessarily aggressively) and professionally following up on a case a therapist makes the importance of his/her referral known and establishes that s/he is truly interested in the client's welfare.

A basic caveat to remember is that although one feels that a report has been made in good faith, the outcome that is desired may not often be realized, leaving a trainee, or even an advanced professional, frustrated and demoralized. Therefore, it is important in the training and supervision of art therapists as supervisors to emphasize that although reporting abuse is a legal issue, there are inevitable emotional issues for the therapist who reports. Discussion of these issues is key to helping supervisees learn how to effectively advocate for their clients whom they suspect to be abused and is just as important as a working knowledge of actual law and procedure.

## Duty-to-Warn

The issue of duty-to-warn historically has it origins from the findings of the Tarasoff case (Tarasoff I, 1974; Tarasoff II, 1976) in which a graduate student at the University of California at Berkeley threatened during a psychotherapy session to kill his girlfriend and then eventually carried out that threat. The therapist did inform police and his supervisor, but did not warn the victim or the victim's family; the therapist was later found negligent. This decision extended the therapists' obligation to clients by stating that therapists not only have a duty to warn, but also a responsibility to protect intended victims.

The Tarasoff decision has become increasingly important in light of the prevalence of domestic violence and AIDS, both issues that might warrant additional obligations on the part of the therapist to warn possible victims. Thus, duty-to-warn is an important topic to discuss with trainees, particularly since supervisors can be held accountable for what their supervisees do or don't do concerning their clients.

## Professional Liability

Professional liability has become an increasing concern for all helping professionals, art therapists included. How to protect oneself in case of a lawsuit by a client, what constitutes malpractice, and professional liability insurance are at the center of these discussions. These issues become extremely important for therapists in private practice, although anyone who works at an agency, clinic, or hospital is not immune to becoming involved in a litigious action. Such negligence as failure to get informed consent, violation of confidentiality, providing services outside the area of one's competence, and dual relationships are a few of the more common causes for malpractice actions (Austin, Moline, & Williams, 1990). Additionally, art therapists have been qualified as expert witnesses (Malchiodi, 1990; Levick, Safran, & Levine, 1990; Cohen-Liebman, 1994; Wirtz, 1994); this recognition of the professional expertise of art therapists also bring with it a greater responsibility for being able to define one's knowledge, skill, experience, training, and education.

Several resources are available to supervisors to introduce trainees to issues surrounding professional liability: general issues of malpractice in psychotherapy (Corey et al, 1993; Austin et al, 1990; Bennett, Bryant, Vandenbos, & Greenwood, 1990); art therapists in private practice (Wirtz, 1994; Wirtz, Sidun, Carrigan, Wadeson, Kennedy, & Marano-Geiser, 1994); expert witness issues (Cohen-Liebman, 1994; Levick, Safran, & Levine, 1990). These articles/presentations are listed in the annotated bibliography at the end of the chapter.

## Strategies for Teaching Ethics and Legal Issues

Aside from reading and discussing articles on ethics and legal issues (a suggested reading list is provided at the end of this chapter), two additional strategies for instructors and supervisors to use with their trainees are included:

### Looking at the Ethical Codes of Other Professionals

It is a given that students and practicing art therapists must be familiar with their own professional code of ethics. Although art therapists are responsible for knowledge of their own code of ethics, examining and discussing the ethical codes of other professions related to art therapy can be helpful in understanding ethics in a general sense and what various professions consider to be ethical (and non-ethical) behavior. Ethical codes of other creative art therapies are a good place to start (see the codes of ethics for AAMT, ADTA, NAPT, NMTA; sources for these are listed in the bibliography at the end of this chapter). The ethical codes of the American Psychological Association, the American Counseling Association, the National Association of Social Workers, the International Association of Play Therapists, and the American Association Marriage & Family Therapy are additional resources. Some training programs and supervisors may use the ethical codes of counselors or marriage and family therapists depending upon the training program or state licensure laws that affect the practice of therapy.

### Using Ethical Dilemmas

Since ethics are really guidelines for professional practice, they are not as clear-cut as one might think. Helping trainees learn to use ethics to inform therapeutic interactions, research, and professionalism is the major point. Therefore, it is important that students be encouraged to think critically and responsibly about ethics and the decision-making process involved in ethics.

Corey, Corey, and Callanan (1993) have written an excellent text on ethics in the helping professions and a great many sample questions and dilemmas are presented that represent the continuum of ethical problems faced in verbal counseling and psychotherapy. Instructors and supervisors will find it easy to generate discussions by using this text and others that are currently available (see Rinas & Clyne-Jackson, 1988; Pope & Vasquez, 1991, for example). However, since art therapy includes the dimensions of visual art and art making, there are some specific circumstances that are somewhat different from those faced by mental health professionals in related fields. Since a great many texts cover ethical questions related to the field of therapy in general, the following examples of ethical dilemmas focus specifically on issues that art therapists face in clinical work.

ETHICAL DILEMMA #1: An art therapist runs several art therapy groups at a local psychiatric hospital where she has worked for three years. Lately, she has realized that there are distinct similarities in the graphic features of the drawings made by the panic disorder clients with whom she has worked. She knows this because she has saved samples of the drawings made by each client who was diagnosed as having panic disorder for the last three years. She wants to share this information with her colleagues in the form of a paper or presentation because she feels that this information could be of great interest to other professionals in the field.

What are some of the ethical problems the art therapist has to examine in utilizing these client's works?

ETHICAL DILEMMA #2: Clients in an art therapy group at an outpatient county mental health agency have worked with the same art therapist for about a year. The group members are all functioning fairly well and include depression, post-traumatic stress, addictions, and anxiety disorders in their diagnoses. The group members are quite excited about the art (drawings, paintings and small sculpture) they have been producing in the group, so much so that they are interested in holding an exhibit of their work at a local church where they could have a reception and also sell their pieces if they wished.

What should the art therapist think about in terms of displaying this groups' art pieces publicly?

ETHICAL DILEMMA #3: An art therapist has been working with a group of children at an outpatient center for children and collecting data on the content of abused children's drawings. He has followed all the appropriate procedures for conducting this research, including obtaining the proper forms and releases. The facility is extremely pleased with his work and wants to highlight his achievements by displaying and selling paintings by the child clients at a fund-raiser to raise money for art therapy programs for abused and neglected children. The executive director in particular thinks this a great idea and is excited that the event will be covered by three large TV stations.

What can this art therapist do to explain ethical problems to his superiors?

The three dilemmas presented are only a starting point for discussion; supervisors who have had many years in the field will easily be able to generate additional ethical 'problems' for their trainees to explore. In addition to dilemmas related specifically to art therapy, supervisors may wish to introduce problems that focus on dual relationships, conflicts between counselor and client values, and group/family work.

Lastly, in addition to presenting actual dilemmas, it is important to give supervisees a framework for ethical decision-making. Corey et al (1993) suggest several steps that may be helpful in dealing with ethical problems, including: clarification of whether the dilemma is ethical or legal, or a combination of both; identification of issues involved; consideration of all possible courses of action; obtaining consultation from knowledgeable clinicians and supervisors. These are all important strategies to instill in trainees and will give them a structure for thinking about the various ethical dilemmas that they will face throughout their professional lives.

For art therapists, personal art making for the purpose of examining one's own beliefs concerning an ethical dilemma is also helpful, especially if the work is shared with an objective colleague or supervisor to assist in one's exploration. Creating an image of one's agency or work setting or using the cartoon strip activity (outlined in Chapter 6) may also be another way to visually explore an ethical dilemma, particularly within a group format.

## Conclusion

Ethics and legal issues are two confusing areas for both trainees and their supervisors. Even the most seasoned professional will be faced on occasion with a situation that can stymie one's own knowledge base in these areas. As with professional issues, it is imperative that a supervisor or instructor have an open mind to the variety of possibilities for interpretation of ethical situations, as well as a responsibility to stay current in laws and regulations governing therapeutic practice.

## References

American Art Therapy Association. (1989). *General standards of practice document*. Mundelein, IL: Author.

American Art Therapy Association. (1990). *Definition of art therapy assessment*. Mundelein, IL: Author.

American Art Therapy Association. (1995). *Ethical standards for art therapists* (includes definition of independent practitioner). Mundelein, IL: Author.

American Counseling Association. (1995). *Standards of practice and ethical standards*. Washington, DC: Author.

American Psychological Association. (1993). *APA code of ethics*. Washington, DC: Author.

Austin, K., Moline, M., & Williams, G. (1990). *Confronting malpractice: Legal and ethical dilemmas in psychotherapy*. Newbury Park, CA: Sage.

Bennett, B. Bryant, B., VandenBos, G. & Greenwood, A. (1990). *Professional liability and risk management.* Washington, DC: American Psychological Association.

Braverman, J. (1995). Retention of treatment records under the new AATA Ethics Standards. *AATA Newsletter, XXVII* (1), 15.

Carrigan, J. (1993). Ethical considerations in a supervisory relationship: A synthesis. *Art Therapy: Journal of the American Art Therapy Association, 10* (3), 130-135.

Cattaneo, M. (1994). Addressing culture and values in the training of art therapists. *Art Therapy: Journal of the American Art Therapy Association, 11*(3), 184-186.

Cattaneo, M., & Gawalek, M. (1994). *Ethical guidelines for core and adjunct faculty: Multiple roles.* Unpublished guidelines from Lesley College Counseling and Expressive Therapies Division.

Cohen-Liebman, M. S. (1994). The art therapist as expert witness in child sexual abuse litigation. *Art Therapy: Journal of the American Art Therapy Association, 11*(4) 260-265.

Corey, G., Corey, M.S., & Callanan, P. (1993). *Issues and ethics in the helping professions:* Pacific Grove, CA: Brooks/Cole.

Kalichman, S.C. (1993). *Mandated reporting of suspected child abuse.* Washington, DC: American Psychological Association.

Levick, M., Safran, D., & Levine, A. (1990). Art therapists as expert witnesses: A judge delivers a precedent-setting decision. *The Arts in Psychotherapy, 17,* 49-53.

Malchiodi, C.A. (1990). *Breaking the silence: Art therapy with children from violent homes.* New York: Brunner/Mazel.

Malchiodi, C.A. (1991). Using drawings in the evaluation of children from violent homes. *Family Violence & Sexual Assault Bulletin, 7* (4), 14-16.

Malchiodi, C.A. (1992). Writing for publication. *Art Therapy: Journal of the American Art Therapy Association, 9* (2), 62- 64.

Malchiodi, C.A. (1994). Certification: In search of accountability. *Art Therapy: Journal of the American Art Therapy Association, 11* (3), 170-172.

Malchiodi, C.A, (1994). Introduction to special section on assessment. *Art Therapy: Journal of the American Art Therapy Association, 11*(1), 104.

Malchiodi, C.A. (1995). Who owns the art ? *Art Therapy: Journal of the American Art Therapy Association, 12* (1), 2-3.

McNiff, S. (1991). Ethics and the autonomy of images. *The Arts in Psychotherapy, 18,* 277-283.

Meriwether, M.H. (1986). Child abuse reporting laws: Time for a change. *Family Law Quarterly, 20,* 141-174.

Moon, C. (1994). What's been left behind: The place of the art product in art therapy. In *Proceedings of the 25th Annual AATA Conference* (p.108), Mundelein, IL: AATA, Inc.

Pope, K.S., & Vasquez, M. (1991). *Ethics in psychotherapy and counseling: A practical guide for psychologists.* San Francisco: Jossey-Bass.

Rinas, J., & Clyne-Jackson, S. (1988). *Professional conduct and legal concerns in mental health practice.* San Mateo, CA: Appleton & Lange.

Ryder, R., & Hepworth, J. (1990). AAMFT ethical code: "Dual relationships." *Journal of Marital & Family Therapy, 16* (2), 127-132.

Spaniol, S. (1990a). Exhibiting art by people with mental illness: Issues, process and principles. *Art Therapy: Journal of the American Art Therapy Association, 2,* 70-78.

Spaniol, S. (1990b). *Organizing exhibitions of art by people with mental illness: A step-by-step manual.* Boston: Center for Psychiatric Rehabilitation, Boston University.

Spaniol, S. (1994). Confidentiality reexamined: Negotiating use of art by clients. *American Journal of Art Therapy, 32* (3), 69-74.

Tarasoff v. Regents of the University of California, 118 Cal. Rptr. 129, 529 P.2D.533. (Cal. 1974).

Tarasoff v. Regents of the University of California, 113 Cal. Rptr. 14, 551, P.2D. 334. (Cal. 1976).

Wadeson, H. (Ed.)(1992). *A guide to conducting art therapy research.* Mundelein, IL: AATA, Inc.

Webster, M. (1994). Legal and ethical issues impacting unlicensed art therapists and their clients in California. *Art Therapy: Journal of the American Art Therapy Association, 11* (4), 278-281.

Wilson, L. (1987). Confidentiality in art therapy: An ethical dilemma. *American Journal of Art Therapy, 25,* 75-80.

Wilson, L., Riley, S., & Wadeson, H. (1984). Art therapy supervision. *Art Therapy: Journal of the American Art Therapy Association, 1* (3), 100-105.

Wirtz, G. (1994). Essential legal issues for art therapists in private practice. *Art Therapy: Journal of the American Art Therapy Association, 11* (4), 293-296.

Wirtz, G., Sidun, N., Carrigan, J., Wadeson, H., Kennedy, S., & Marano-Geiser, R. (1994). *Legal issues: Can art therapists stand alone?* Denver, CO: National Audio Video tape # 58-149.

## Annotated Bibliography on Ethics & Legal Issues for Art Therapists

American Psychological Association. (1982). *Ethical principles in the conduct of research with human subjects.* Washington, DC: Author. This is a standard text and is a universally accepted guide to the ethics of research. Although the AATA ethical code is similar to the APA tenets concerning research, this document delineates the responsibilities of the investigator.

Braverman, J. (1995). Retention of treatment records under the new AATA Ethics Standards. *AATA Newsletter, XXVII (1)*, 15. This article covers some of the legal issues involved in retention and storage of client art (The specific issue of the newsletter is available from the AATA national office).

Cattaneo, M. (1994). Addressing culture and values in the training of art therapists. *Art Therapy: Journal of the American Art Therapy Association, 11*(3), 184-186. The author discusses the importance of including multicultural and gender issues in the training of art therapy students at the graduate level.

Cohen-Liebman, M. S. (1994). The art therapist as expert witness in child sexual abuse litigation. *Art Therapy: Journal of the American Art Therapy Association, 11*(4) 260-265. One of very few articles specifically for art therapists that addresses legal aspects of being an expert witness; Cohen-Liebman's piece is part of a larger, more comprehensive graduate thesis on the subject.

Corey, G., Corey, M.S., & Callanan, P. (1993). *Issues and ethics in the helping professions.* Pacific Grove, CA: Brooks/Cole. Standard text that articulately delineates what every therapist should know in areas of ethics, legal matters, and professional issues.

Kalichman, S.C. (1993). *Mandated reporting of suspected child abuse.* Washington, DC: American Psychological Association. This book provides up-to-date information on reporting of suspected child abuse and neglect; real bonuses are the compilation of reporting laws in all fifty states and the resource list of child abuse/neglect agencies across the country.

Malchiodi, C.A. (1991). Using drawings in the evaluation of children from violent homes. *Family Violence & Sexual Assault Bulletin, 7* (3), 14-16. This short article may be helpful to introduce ethical issues of using art expression in the assessment of children to non-art therapists. The need for competency, obtaining current information on research, and understanding the child client's perspective are emphasized.

Malchiodi, C.A. (1995). Who owns the art? *Art Therapy: Journal of the American Art Therapy Association, 12* (1), 2-3. A discussion of the ethical issues in the retention of client art as part of medical treatment records and the unique dilemmas that face art therapists in this area.

McNiff, S. (1991). Ethics and the autonomy of images. *The Arts in Psychotherapy, 18*, 277-283. Philosophical and impassioned discussion of the need for respect for clients' images created in art therapy.

Spaniol, S. (1990a). Exhibiting art by people with mental illness: Issues, process and principles. *Art Therapy: Journal of the American Art Therapy Association, 2*, 70-78. Through this article and a manual (see next entry), Spaniol identifies ethical, legal and personal aspects in the exhibition of client art and presents clearly defined guidelines for how to set up an exhibit from start to finish.

Spaniol, S. (1990b). *Organizing exhibitions of art by people with mental illness: A step-by-step manual.* Boston: Center for Psychiatric Rehabilitation, Boston University.

Wilson, L. (1987). Confidentiality in art therapy: An ethical dilemma. *American Journal of Art Therapy, 25*, 75-80. One of very few articles written on the unique aspects of confidentiality in art therapy.

Wirtz, G. (1994). Essential legal issues for art therapists in private practice. *Art Therapy: Journal of the American Art Therapy Association, 11* (4), 293-296. This article provides some basic caveats and considerations in establishing a private art therapy practice, with an emphasis on liability and malpractice issues.

Wirtz, G., Sidun, N., Carrigan, J., Wadeson, H., Kennedy, S., & Marano-Geiser, R. (1994). *Legal issues: Can art therapists stand alone?* Denver, CO: National Audio Video tape # 58-149. Four art therapists and a lawyer discuss various topics relating to law and ethics and provide suggestions to avoid malpractice or other legal problems.

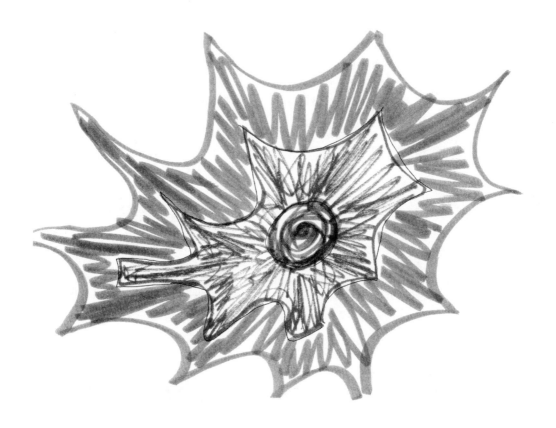

Supervision... an explosion of anxieties, a core of information.

# CHAPTER FOURTEEN

## Exposure and the Consequences of Legal Liability in Art Therapy Training and Supervision
by Linda Randlett Kollar

There is no question that the training and education of the intern must include substantive material related to ethics and legal issues which are inextricably interwoven into the therapeutic process. Questions are constantly raised about legal and ethical issues, such as statutory reporting duties, confidentiality, and dual relationships, which must be addressed in supervision. Consequently, any competent supervisor must be armed with intimate knowledge about the content of the relevant ethical codes and the statutory mandates of the profession.

Beyond the substantive knowledge of the ethical and legal aspects of the profession, however, remains an understanding of liability and the consequences for the supervisor and trainee for a failure to adhere to their legal and ethical duties. In my practice as an attorney, I represent professionals in the fields of psychiatry, psychology, social work, and counseling. On uncountable occasions, I have heard the stunned, quivering voice of a seasoned therapist on the other end of the telephone announcing that they are the subject of an investigation by the licensing board, the police, or they have just received a summons and complaint naming them as a defendant. When the

*This chapter is contributed by Linda Randlett Kollar, attorney and partner of the Los Angeles based firm of Weinhart and Riley. Ms. Kollar's practice includes the representation of professionals in health and health-related fields.*

211

case involves supervision, I am frequently told that the therapist remembers the supervisee but they know nothing about the underlying case. There are questions such as: Am I really being held accountable for the acts of a trainee when I, the supervisor, had no knowledge of the alleged activities? What about the fact that all of these acts allegedly took place many years ago? Is there some basis for direct liability on grounds of improper supervision? Is my license to practice at risk? What are the potential consequences?

The current climate of escalated claims of malpractice against health professionals is one that makes these questions and other related subjects particularly ripe for inquiry. We are living in a litigious society in which therapists have not emerged unscathed and like many others in the healing arts, therapists have felt the chilling effects of malpractice suits. Furthermore, we are living in a society in which our government seeks to closely regulate all professionals through the establishment of various licensing boards.

This chapter will survey the basis for legal liability in the context of supervision, the scope of exposure based on the supervisor/trainee relationship, the forum for legal action, and, finally some suggestions for 'risk' management by incorporating legal issues into the art therapy practice.

While this information is for the most part generic as applied to all theories or models of supervision and all therapeutic modalities, where appropriate, specific reference is made to application in the art therapy context. This information is imparted not to make therapists lawyers, but to enhance the enjoyment of the practice by making the law a working partner. The goal must be for the therapist to practice within the law while balancing professional and moral duties.

## The Scope of Liability

Legal liability arises within the scope of the supervisor/trainee relationship either directly or vicariously.

### Direct Liability

One way in which the supervisor may be held directly liable to both clients and trainees is a result of a breach or failure to fulfill the statutory requirements for licensure. Many states, for example, within their licensure acts, set forth with great specificity the minimum standards for licensure and concurrently the duties and responsibilities of the supervisor and supervisee. A state's business and professions code may enumerate all of the responsibilities of the supervisor, including a duty to be responsible for ensuring the extent, kind, and quality of counseling performed and for assuring the licensure board that all laws, rules, and regulations governing the practice are enforced.

Furthermore, the regulations may set forth the number of hours of supervision that are required for licensure, along with the setting in which an intern may be supervised, and notification requirements for reporting hours to the board (see for example, California Business and Professions Code Sections 4980 et seq.). Any deviation from these mandates could result in claims of negligence and/or unprofessional conduct.

Charges of direct liability may also be alleged on grounds of 'negligent' supervision if the supervisor has been derelict in the supervision of the trainee. Such claims are most likely to occur when there has been a breach of the aforementioned statutory duties or may be raised under a theory that ethical guidelines have not been adhered to, thereby giving rise to unprofessional conduct. Ethical guidelines such as those promulgated for art therapists by the American Art Therapy Association provide that the supervisor is responsible for the planning, course, and outcome of the supervisee's work (AATA, Ethical Standards for Art Therapists). Direct liability could occur under these guidelines, for example, if the supervisor gave the trainee inappropriate advice regarding treatment and the trainee carried it out to the patient's detriment (Dooley, 1977). Direct liability could also accrue if the supervisor failed to listen carefully to the trainee's comments about the client, failed to comprehend the client's needs, or generally failed to carry out his or her supervisory duties. The supervisor could be liable if he gave a task to a trainee who was inadequately trained in that the supervisor is expected to know the level of skill of his supervisees (Harrar, VandeCreek & Knapp, 1990).

Marilyn, a therapist who had done supervision for 17 years, was caught completely off guard when she received a call from the state licensing board that she had not paid her professional fees for renewal of her license. While this was an innocent mistake, the board's position was that: 1) she was practicing without a license (grounds for revocation of her license); and 2) none of the hours that her students had accrued during the three months she was unlicensed would count toward their education or statutory requirements for a license. Moreover, one of her trainees was furious and threatening to sue. This true story elaborates the potential for direct liability based on the duty of the supervisor to adhere to all statutory requirements of the profession. Failure to do so in this case put at risk Marilyn's license and a potential lawsuit resulting from her negligence.

### Dual Relationship

One cannot address the issue of direct liability without a discussion of the potential for a dual relationship between supervisor and trainee. A dual relationship is one in which there are two (or more) distinct kinds of relationships with the same person (Tomm, 1993).

There is no doubt that dual relationships form the major basis of licensing disciplinary actions, malpractice suits, and ethical complaints. The code of ethics of the American Association of Marriage and Family Therapy expressly defines dual relationships to be avoided by supervisors. In addition to forbidding sexual involvement, the code enjoins therapists from doing business or maintaining close personal relationships with supervisees, students, or employees; nor are therapists to provide therapy to students, employees, or supervisees (American Association for Marriage and Family Therapy, 1991). The American Art Therapy Association Code of Ethics also addresses dual relationships but in a more general way, and expressly forbids a supervisor from engaging in therapy with students or supervisees (AATA, Ethical Standards for Art Therapists).

The argument against engaging in dual relationships because of the potential for disaster is expressed by Michele Bograd (1993) as follows:

> "The basic argument against dual relationships goes something like this: The hierarchical nature of the therapist/patient or teacher/student relationship, which seems a necessary aspect of the professional encounter, undermines truly equal consent to the nonprofessional connection. Even an ethical practitioner may unconsciously exploit or damage clients or students, who are inherently vulnerable in the relationship. Once the clarity of professional boundaries has been muddied, there is good chance for confusion, disappointment and disillusionment on both sides." (p. 8)

Serious conflicts, ripe for subjecting the therapist to liability, are bound to occur if the supervisor and trainee pursue a dual relationship, especially one that resolves in sexual intimacy during professional training. Included in this admonition is the situation in which the supervisor provides therapy to the supervisee; this is never ethical (Borys & Pope 1989).

### Vicarious Liability

Vicarious liability is the doctrine that provides that a supervisor, though personally innocent, will be liable for the negligence of a supervisee for the acts committed within the scope of their duties. In the case of the supervisor/ trainee relationship, such liability is imputed because the persons involved stand in such a relationship to each other that it can be said that one acted through the control of the other (46 Cal.Jur. 3d).

Since most trainees are also employees of the supervisor, the legal doctrine of respondeat superior may be invoked to hold supervisors liable for the actions of their employees/trainees. In some states, such as California, the

Business and Professions Code mandates that the supervisee must be an employee, "Interns and trainees may only perform services as employees and not independent contractors" (California Business & Profession Code Section 1833(d)(3)). The distinction between employee and independent contractor is important because as independent contractors the potential for imputed or vicarious liability would be significantly lessened. Under the doctrine of respondeat superior, however, an employer is not only vicariously liable for the negligence of his employees but, in some instances, employers have been held liable for the willful, malicious, or even criminal acts of an employee.

Carol was outraged and horrified when the state board named her in an accusation and sought revocation of her clinical social work license on grounds that she had supervised a trainee who had engaged in a sexual relationship with a client. The intimate relationship between the supervisee and client was a complete surprise to Carol. The intern had never mentioned this relationship when they discussed the case and there were no hints of the egregious impropriety. Carol could demonstrate that she had not been negligent in her supervision. She had fulfilled the requirements mandated both by her agency and the statutes. However, under a theory of vicarious liability, Carol, although not directly guilty of any negligence, would be placed in the shoes of her supervisee and found equally culpable for the supervisee's breach of both ethical and statutory duties, by engaging in a dual relationship.

This expanded exposure of the supervisor resulting from vicarious liability makes clear that the supervisor must assume final responsibility for the client (Harrar, VandeCreek & Knapp, 1990). Clearly, the stakes are too high and the risk too great for the supervisor not to be familiar with each case of every supervisee (Cormier & Bernard, 1982).

## The Standard of Care

The law presumes and holds all therapists to a standard of reasonable care when dealing with clients (Simon, 1992). The essence of any legal claim against a health professional will be testimony which shall determine the degree and skill and required learning necessary in treating a patient that is customarily applied in treating a patient similarly afflicted in the same community and under the same circumstances. This has been defined as the "standard of reasonable care." (36 Cal.Jur.3d) A succinct definition of the standard of reasonableness in the case of a physician, which is applicable to therapists, has been described as follows:

"In the absence of a special contract, a physician or surgeon is not required to exercise extraordinary skill and care or the highest degree of skill and care possible; but as a general rule, he (or she) is only required to possess and exercise the degree of skill and learning ordinarily possessed and exercised, under similar circumstances, by the members of his (or her) profession in good standing, and to use ordinary and reasonable care and diligence, and his (or her) best judgment, in the application of his (or her) skill to the case." (Simon, 1993, p. 4)

The trainee is held to the same standard of care as the licensed professional (Harrar, VandeCreek & Knapp, 1990). It is therefore not a defense that the trainee was 'inexperienced' or did not have sufficient training and therefore acted negligently or failed to fulfill a mandated duty.

In litigation, both prosecutors, plaintiffs, and defendants will establish the standard of care by expert testimony. Experts will give evidence of their credentials as established practitioners and their credibility to testify, as being familiar with the community, with the statutes, literature, and applicable ethical codes related to their practice.

The use of ethical codes to determine the standard of care is controversial. The controversy is whether an ethical code is aspirational or whether it is a statement of expectations. The American Art Therapy Association's ethical code is preluded by the following language:

The board of directors of the American Art Therapy Association (AATA) hereby promulgate, pursuant to Article 8, Sections 1, 2, and 3 of the Association By-Laws, a revised code of ethical standards for art therapists. Members of AATA abide by these standards and by applicable state laws and regulations governing the conduct of art therapists and any additional license or certification which the art therapist holds (AATA, Ethical Standards for Art Therapists, 1995).

This language and language similar in other and related disciplines arguably implies that membership in the AATA establishes these standards as mandatory for ethical practice by the association's members. In my experience, ethical codes of recognized professional associations are admitted into evidence for purposes of establishing the standard of care.

Because the standard of care forms the grounds for any charge of unprofessional conduct, it is imperative that the practitioner keep abreast of changes in ethical codes, the literature of the practice, and accepted modalities of treatment. Examples of standard or care issues related to art therapy that may be the subject of a claim of 'unprofessional' conduct and for which there are no clear guidelines are whether the duties related to confidentiality are breached when art is anonymously exhibited with permission in a public place where friends or family may recognize the work or issues about the obligations of the therapist in abandoning work when therapy has terminated.

Organizations of professionals such as the American Art Therapy Association are important vehicles for professionals to keep abreast of issues related to standard of care within their field and for each therapist to implement conservative practices. Good defensive practices rooted in the best conservative traditions are quintessential to survival in our litigious environment. Some of these defensive practices include careful documentation and appropriate consultation which, are good clinical practice on behalf of the patient and also provide a shield against litigation.

## The Forum

Claims for liability for failure to perform within the standard of care may result in a complaint in civil court for malpractice, a criminal complaint, an accusation from the licensing board, and, some professional associations may initiate a peer review.

### Malpractice

The most common example of a legal action against a practitioner is for malpractice in which the plaintiff seeks compensation for alleged damages that have occurred. The fundamental concept underlying a malpractice suit is generally negligence. In the world of health care, negligence is best described as "doing something that he or she should not have done (commission) or omitting to do something that he or she should have done (omission)" (Simon, 1993, p. 3). A substantial deviation from the standard of care resulting in substandard conduct which is generally claimed to be outrageous may constitute "gross negligence". The fundamental elements of a prima facia case for malpractice are:

1) The establishment of a duty of care—the law must recognize a relationship which creates rights and duties for all parties. For example, the relationship giving rise to such a duty is that of supervisor and trainee which creates a legal duty to both clients and trainees;

2) A breach or deviation from the standard of care—the creation of the duty generates the promise that the supervisor will exercise reasonable care. An elaborated definition of the standard of care within the practice is found earlier in this chapter;

3) Proof of resulting damage to the plaintiff—damages are generally awarded that are commensurate with the extent of the injury sustained. There are generally three types of damages: compensatory, nominal and punitive. In a malpractice action, compensatory damages are normally awarded. These damages should amount to compensation to replace and restore the loss or injury to the plaintiff. Punitive damages will only be awarded when the defendant's conduct is considered willful, wanton, malicious or reckless. Finally, nominal damages are awarded when plaintiff suffered no actual harm or loss, but only a technical injury to their legal right; and

4) Proof that the damage occurred directly as a result of deviation from the standard of care—it is relevant to determine whether the plaintiff has pre-existing injuries and that whether all of the damages alleged are the result of the breach.

Civil claims might also be alleged on other causes of action, typically for intentional acts. An intentional "tort" is a willful malicious wrongdoing. For example, sexual misconduct, offensive touching, or treating a patient without consent, might be construed to be acts of intentional misconduct.

The major areas of liability brought for malpractice against a therapist are 1) claims of harm resulting from a dual relationship with a patient or the supervisee (including sexual misconduct), 2) breach of reporting duties, 3) failure to get informed consent, and 4) breach of confidentiality.

Within the scheme of the supervisor/supervisee relationship, the risk of liability is generally found in issues related to informed consent and confidentiality. Not only must informed consent be imparted to the patient so that they may make informed choices related to treatment, but the patient must be made fully aware that the therapist they are seeing is a trainee and that the trainee is meeting on a regular basis for supervisorial sessions. Since by virtue of supervision, supervisors have a relationship with the client whom a trainee is counseling, it is important that the client be informed of that relationship in all details (Borders & Leddick, 1987).

Supervisors must make sure that clients are fully informed about the limits of confidentiality, including those situations in which supervisors have a duty to warn or to protect. Secondly, the client should be informed that supervisors will be meeting regularly with their supervisees and the client's case may be discussed in group supervision meetings with other trainees (Corey, Corey & Callanan, 1993).

Despite what seems to be unfettered exposure for liability, it should be clearly understood that therapists should not, as a matter of law, be held liable for mere mistakes or the failure to effect a 'cure' (Simon, 1993). Furthermore, innovations in treatment should be distinguished from a deviation from the requisite standard of care. Indeed, over 450 types of therapy have been identified and innovation is a commonly recognized requisite in treating difficult patients. However, while a therapist should not be held liable when his or her treatment methods differ from those of main stream therapy, the therapist in today's litigation climate is well advised that they may have to defend their practice if they choose such deviations in treatment.

### Criminal Complaints

Some conduct may result in a criminal complaint against the therapist.

Most notably, in some states the failure of a therapist to report child abuse may bring with it criminal sanctions including a fine and incarceration. Other duties which may result in criminal liability are insurance (billing), fraud or medicare or medicaid fraud. Sexual misconduct has also been known to result in charges of rape or sexual assault.

### Licensure Board Actions

The fundamental purpose of state licensing boards is to protect the consumer from practitioners who are not competent and who present a risk to the public's welfare.

At issue in a disciplinary action brought by a state licensing board is the professional's right to practice his or her profession. The stakes are high and could wipe out a lifetime of work. Most therapists are shocked to learn that once such a proceeding is begun, most administrative law forums provide limited rights for the accused and few procedural protections.

In California, for example, a licensee, if he does not testify in his own behalf, can be called in the rebuttal case by the board (California Government Code Section 11513(b)). This is unlike a criminal case in which a defendant cannot be compelled to testify against himself and does not at any point have to take the stand.

Additionally, in most board actions, even though criminal statutes may be part of the charges and the conduct may be the same as what would be involved in a criminal case, the standard of proof is only by clear and convincing proof to a reasonable certainty (see Ettinger v. Board of Medical Quality Assurance, 135 Cal.App.3d 853, 185 Cal.Rptr. 601 (1982)). In a criminal case, charges must be proven beyond a reasonable doubt, a much higher standard than "proof to a reasonable certainty".

Most shockingly, there are no statutes of limitation. A patient may wait five, ten, or twenty years to file a complaint with the board. With civil actions for professional malpractice, the statute of limitations is generally one year. The prejudice a respondent faces when there is no statute of limitations is substantial. Witnesses may have disappeared and memories faded. In the field of psychotherapy, modalities of treatment change significantly over the years. Practices accepted in the 1960s and 1970s are clearly not within the standards of today's care. For a licensing board to challenge the accused therapist for practices of the 60's and 70's in the 1990's and apply today's standard of care is patently unjust.

The greatest inequity arises in those states where after an administrative hearing and a decision has been rendered by an administrative law judge, the board is then free to accept, modify, or reject the administrative law judge's decision (California Government Code Section 11517(c)). Finally, in board actions, no matter how disturbed the claimant may be, there is no device to obtain any discovery of that claimant's current mental condition.

While there are many grass roots professional organizations, both of practitioners and attorneys who are seeking to change these unjust aspects of the administrative law process, the foregoing represents the current state of due process for the licensee.

### Peer Review

Some professional organizations, upon receiving a complaint regarding a member, will institute peer review and make an independent determination about whether the therapist should be sanctioned for unprofessional conduct by that organization.

### Interaction

Do not be so naive as to believe that only one of the foregoing consequences may result from any given alleged violation of your legal and ethical duties.

As a practical matter, a complaint arising in one forum will usually be brought in one or two of the others. For example, a complaint for malpractice may be reported to the licensure board and to a professional organization by the plaintiff, counsel, or even through media publicity. The board may issue an accusation and the professional organization may proceed with peer review. The therapist is then faced with defending a complaint in civil court, an accusation in the administrative law forum, and a peer review on terms and conditions of their professional association. All of these actions may take place concurrently, much to the therapist's financial and emotional drain.

## Risk Management - Integrating The Law Into Practice

Practicing defensively creates within itself many ethical dilemmas for the therapist. As one author has suggested, defensive practice comes in two forms: positive and negative (Simon, 1993).

The negative practice results from a "climate of fear" and has been described by one therapist as follows:

"Across the country a climate of fear is developing among clinical psychologists. They are afraid to be inventive or creative in their treatments lest their approach be viewed as outside the 'standard of practice'. They are unwilling to take on psychological assistants, as that would increase their legal exposure. They are afraid to touch their clients, even simply to reassure or comfort. At malpractice prevention workshops, clinicians are advised not to see borderline or multiple personality character disorders. Clinicians use case notes to protect themselves rather than to further their clinical understanding. They are increasingly suggesting consultations with other health care providers as a way of distributing responsibility for a diagnosis or procedure. They are increasingly urging medication as a therapeutic solution. Suffering under the burden of fear and hyper-caution clinicians are experiencing a chilling effect in the way they conduct psychotherapy. Meanwhile, in this adversarial atmosphere, all consumers are not receiving proper care.

Why is this happening? Because there has been a dramatic increase in malpractice civil suits against psychologists. Furthermore, there has been a remarkable increase in the number of complaints filed with licensing boards against practitioners. For example, in California, by the end of June 1993, the board of psychology received twice as many complaints as it had during the previous year. Complaints are filed by 'consumers' (i.e., patients), relatives of patients, fellow colleagues and members of other disciplines. In addition, malpractice carriers are required to report settlements to the appropriate licensing board(s)." (Sherven, 1994, p. 48)

The following are not exclusive, but are some suggestions for structuring an effective practice that encompasses the tension between clinical and legal requirements in establishing a positive defense practice:

1) Keep and maintain adequate clinical records. The existence of critical information may be reviewed by an expert and an opinion can be obtained that the practitioner has met the standard of care.

2) Keep all documents authorized by the patient. Nothing can be more persuasive than a production in the patient's own handwriting.

3) Document the client's informed consent to both treatment and an understanding that a trainee will be consulting with a supervisor.

4) Be clear on statutorily required reporting duties and how they interface with issues of confidentiality. Remember that even when statutes require a reporting, disclosure may involve some discretionary acts on behalf of the therapist.

5) Use supervision or consult a colleague when ethical decisions seem unresolvable or to regain a perspective when issues arise.

6) Consider corroborating any diagnosis with clinical testing, including an MMPI as a method of supporting clinical impressions.

7) If progressive boundary violations occur between therapist and patient, the patient should be referred out. In the instance of supervisor/supervisee boundary violations, supervision should be terminated.

8) Supervisors should take the responsibility of knowing about every case in supervision. A competent supervisor must be intimately familiar with statutory duties, including all licensure duties, and obligations of both the supervisor and supervisee.

9) Keep updated on all changes in the appropriate discipline ethical codes through periodicals and association in professional organizations.

## Conclusion

Any therapist who is involved in supervision must be conscious of the exposure for legal liability and the consequences of criminal, civil, and administrative penalties. As a supervisor, the exposure is broadened on theories of vicarious liability and respondeat superior.

Notwithstanding this potential for liability, if a clinician has a good working knowledge of the relevant legal requirements governing the professional practice and implements strategies for a positive defense practice, the law will be a partner to overcoming the climate of fear posed by our litigious society.

## References

American Art Therapy Association (1995). *Ethical standards for art therapists.* Mundelein, Il: Author.

American Association of Marriage and Family Therapists. (1991). *AAMFT Code of Ethics.* Washington, D.C.: Author.

Bogard, M. (1993). The duel over dual relationships. *The California Therapist, 5*(1), 7-19

Borders, L.D. & Leddick, G.R. (1987). *Handbook of counseling supervision.* Alexandria, VA: Association for Counselor Education and Supervision.

Borys, D.S. and Pope, K.S. (1989). Dual relationships between therapist and client: A national study of psychologists, psychiatrists, and social workers. *Professional Psychology: Research and Practice, 20*(5), 283-293.

Corey, C., Corey, M.S. & Callanan, D. (1993). *Issues and ethics in the helping profession.* Pacific Grove, CA: Brooks/Cole.

Cormier, L.S. & Bernard, J.M. (1982). Ethical and legal responsibilities of clinical supervisors. *Personnel and Guidance Journal, 60*(8), 486-490.

Dooley, J.A. (1977). *Modern tort law: Liability and litigation (Vol. 2).* Chicago, Il: Callaghan.

Harrar, W.K., VandeCreek, L. & Knapp, S. (1990). Ethical and legal aspects of clinical supervision. *Professional Psychology: Research & Practice, 21*(1), 37-41.

Sherven, J. (1994). Guilty until proven innocent. *The Independent Practitioner, Division 42 of the American Psychological Association, 14*(2), 48-50.

Simon, R. I. (1992). *Psychiatry and law for clinicians.* Washington, D.C.: American Psychiatric Press.

Tomm, K. (1993). The ethics of dual relationships. *The California Therapist, 5*(1), 7-19.

California Government Code.

California Business & Professional Code.

46 Cal.Jur.3d. (1978). Negligence, 256-258.

36 Cal.Jur.3d. (1978). *Healing Arts and Institutions*, 350-362.

Ettinger v. Board of Medical Quality Assurance, 135 Cal.App.3d.853, 185 Cal.Rptr.601 (1982)

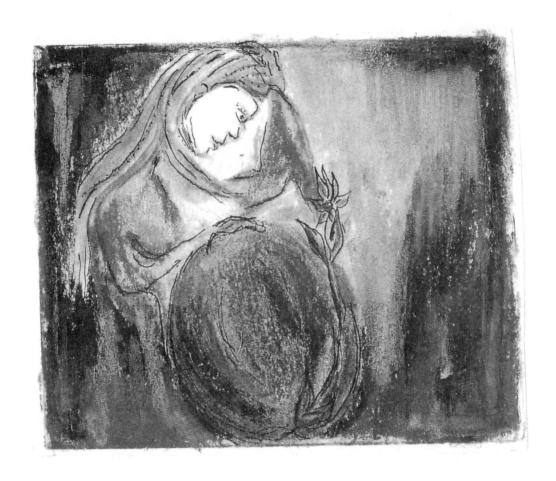

Supervision

# CHAPTER FIFTEEN

## Writing for Professional Publications
by Cathy A. Malchiodi

Professional and scholarly writing is a topic that should be discussed in the training and supervision of art therapists. Although this may seem like more of an academic issue rather than a supervisory one, often supervisors or supervision seminar instructors at the graduate level are asked to advise their supervisees on how to prepare a paper for publication or presentation. Also, clear and effective writing is certainly essential in the job market and will continue to be necessary throughout one's career. With the continued emphasis on communication skills and the need for articulate communication of the value of art therapy, writing is a professional skill that cannot be ignored in the training of students.

As an art therapy educator and supervisor I have seen a great deal of poorly written communication from students and supervisees. Understandably, students who come to the profession from an art or humanities background are often at a disadvantage in the area of technical writing. Supervisors and instructors are often not knowledgeable about the basics of scholarly writing, particularly how to write effectively about clinical, methodological, and theoretical issues. As role models for students and supervisees, supervisors and instructors bear at least some responsibility for this area of learning.

This brief chapter will not be able to address all the various attributes of good writing; there are many resources that describe these concepts (some of which are described in the resource list at the end of this chapter). Also, it is not for the supervisor, or, for that matter, the graduate-level instructor to teach a student or supervisee how to write; these are skills that for the most part, should be acquired before graduate level training begins. What I am suggesting, however, is that supervisors and instructors have a basic understanding of scholarly writing in order to assist students in developing professional, technical, and ethical skills in this area.

## Writing for Scholarly Publications

Many students and supervisees will have good ideas for scholarly papers, but often have no idea of how to get started and what is required to write for publication. They may even attempt a submission to a journal of a paper that an instructor or supervisor has praised, only to be flatly rejected because of the style, format, lack of editing, or lack of references. They also generally have no idea of how to interact with professional journals, editors, or the peer review process, nor do they understand that journals often receive a great many submissions that must either be rejected or must undergo substantial revisions before publication. Considering the time and effort it takes to write an article for a journal or other peer-reviewed publication, it is important to carefully consider the following aspects in developing and finalizing a manuscript for submission.

When submitting a manuscript to most publications, it is extremely important for all prospective authors to first pay close attention to the guidelines for authors; these are generally listed in the front or back of a journal. Most journals that art therapists will submit manuscripts to use the publication guidelines for the American Psychological Association (1994, 4th ed.). Oversights such as lack of adherence to style and format in both the body of the text and references will cause the submission to be immediately rejected, or at the very least, slow down the review process and possible publication of a manuscript. A great many manuscripts present interesting and thoughtful information, but have not met the simple standards outlined and are therefore returned to the author without review. Often these are pieces that have some potential, but the author has not taken the time to follow guidelines for submission, the result being flat rejection.

Another common problem is that authors, especially first-time writers, often neglect to identify how they specifically derived their information. In scholarly writing, it is imperative to define how observations were made and conclusions drawn. In general, there are two categories of observations when writing about art therapy: clinical observations and observations made as the result of definable research methodology. Clinical observations are generally those made in the course of treatment of a client and involve personal views and speculations about what has transpired. There is nothing particularly wrong with clinical observations, although it is likely that such observations are less robust than those conclusions drawn from well-designed and carefully executed research. They occur most frequently in narrative case research which has been a traditional staple of art therapy writing. There are, as many in this profession are aware, significant drawbacks to the narrative case study approach (Malchiodi, 1992; Rosal, 1989) and many journals discourage case studies unless a particular methodology is utilized.

Research observations are derived from a carefully constructed research study. In order to accurately communicate the implications of research observations, the specific research methodology used must be accurately described so that the reader is fully informed about how the author arrived at his/her conclusions. Again, journal guidelines for submission and the APA guidelines for publication will describe the format and content of how to present research methodology. However, what is most important is that the author identify the origin of observations so that the reader is fully cognizant of the manner in which the author derived any conclusions; this will also clarify to the reviewers of the paper how the author derived his/her thoughts and ideas.

One of the greatest dangers that an author confronts when writing a scholarly paper is that the final manuscript may be only a collection of appropriate quotations and really nothing of his/her own. Many a student paper and some doctoral and masters theses have succumbed to this practice. To avoid this over reliance on quoted material, a rule of thumb when using quotations is to always move on from the quotation and continue the paragraph by developing the idea presented in the quote. By forcing a response to the quote, the author begins a dialogue with the information. This process also naturally leads to a synthesis of ideas, both those from the quoted source and the author's own developing arguments.

Lastly, it is particularly important in scholarly writing to be critical. This does not mean that an author has to be cruel in order to make a point, but he or she needs to ask questions about what others have written. On one level, being critical means taking nothing for granted, e.g. not believing things because an authority figure says so or because it is in print. It also refers to the capacity to thoughtfully analyze the ideas, statements, and premises of others. This is particularly important in the field of art therapy where many of our basic theories and methodologies are still subject to debate, require clarification, or need further substantiation.

## Importance of a Literature Review

A thorough and accurate literature review is extremely important to building an argument particularly if the article is theoretically based, and is a necessity if extending some area of research. Often manuscripts are returned to authors because there are obvious gaps in citations of current literature. Undoubtedly, a literature review is time-consuming, and a good reference library with a current collection of periodicals and dissertation abstracts must be consulted. Often a computer search is also necessary; access to library CD-ROM databases and computer on-line services can provide periodical, dissertation abstracts, and other references. It is also important to look closely at what has been published during the last five years, particularly if you are reviewing literature relevant to research.

In some ways, a literature review is often more difficult in the field of art therapy than in other disciplines. First, an author has to sift through references in a variety of subjects such as social and behavioral sciences, medicine, psychiatry, visual art, art education, special education, and anthropology, depending on the theme of the manuscript. This will often involve looking at material in several different databases and perhaps even different libraries. Also, much of the literature in art therapy journals has yet to be referenced in many of the major databases, so hand searches of journal issues are often required for an accurate overview.

Additionally, much of the art therapy knowledge base has been part of oral history at the Annual AATA Conferences where current professional issues, methodology, and theory have been discussed and debated over the years. Research findings are often presented in this forum, many of which have not been published in any professional journal, book, or source other than self-published manuals. The latter is difficult for most individuals to obtain because they are generally only available directly from the author(s) and are not referenced for library purposes. Much of the information presented at the AATA conferences may only be available on audio tape or in the annual Proceedings in which short papers and synopses of presentations have been published; since the mid 1980's, only abstracts have been published. Therefore, due to the variety of sources, it takes a special effort to explore what has already been discussed, developed, or distilled in our professional field.

As our profession continues to expand and become more visible, it is essential for authors to be aware of what is going on in the world outside art therapy. It is obvious that others are investigating the use and meaning of art in therapy and that their perspectives are important in defining our own. With the rapid advancement of knowledge in so many disciplines that are related to art therapy, it may seem impossible to stay abreast of current trends and developments that affect our field. However, one way to keep informed is to regularly consult professionals outside art therapy or, at the very least, peruse their professional journals. In this way, an author can at least get a *feel* for what is currently being debated or investigated and will know where to look for necessary information to develop ideas for theoretical, methodological, or research papers.

## Writing an Abstract

A good way to help students get experience in developing written material for eventual publication is to assign the writing of an abstract of research or clinical work. An abstract is a short piece, usually one page or less, describing a proposed research project, a theoretical or clinical presentation. It generally contains a concise literature review, a hypothesis (if research), goals, and objectives of the proposed project, and what the reader or audience will learn from the paper or presentation. An abstract should be able to stand alone as a brief description of the paper, research, or proposed presentation.

Abstracts are used in the review process for acceptance of presentations at professional conferences. For example, the American Art Therapy Association and other professional associations that put out calls for papers provide specific guidelines for submission and style of abstracts. Often agencies and foundations request abstracts in order to preview requests for grant monies; although they are not required by all sponsors, it is advisable to include an abstract with a grant proposal as it quickly and effectively summarizes a request to reviewers. Most journals require that an abstract be included along with the submission of an article; in this situation, the abstract is used for referencing purposes by databases. Researchers often decide on the basis of an abstract whether to read an entire article, so it is important to know how to write one effectively.

Writing an abstract requires that the person narrow his/her focus of the paper or presentation and conduct a literature search to determine what has been contributed on the topic in the past. Questions to ask oneself when writing an abstract include:

- In one sentence, what is the purpose of this paper or presentation?
- What will the scope of the presentation include?
- What are the sources used to support the purpose (personal experiences, articles, books, etc.)?
- What are the conclusions or implications of the paper or presentation?

Each year the AATA publishes proceedings of its annual conferences which includes the abstracts of peer-reviewed, accepted papers, panels, and workshops. Although the abstracts vary greatly in quality and clarity, this is a good place to start to familiarize oneself with what information is included in an abstract. Journal articles (art therapy or related fields such as psychology or counseling) are another source of sample abstracts and are especially good to review when writing an abstract for submission of an article.

## The Ethics of Writing About Clients

Writing about art therapy often includes writing about clients, especially when describing a clinical application of our field. It is also very easy to slip into discussing our clients as part of larger clinical or research papers or presentations. It is natural to illustrate theoretical and methodological concepts with a client description and a well-presented client case is always of interest to readers and/or the audience. However, it is often harder to remember and honor the responsibilities incumbent upon us when discussing a client's history, verbal expression, and art products in presenting clinical or research data.

Some standard ethical caveats govern the use of client history, observations, and communications (verbal and artistic) in writing. Confidentiality is one of the most important aspects; in most cases, it is unethical to reveal a client's identity. This usually means the use of a pseudonym to disguise the person's name and an effort to camouflage other identifying characteristics. Additionally, written permission to discuss a client's history and art expressions should be obtained before including this information in an article, not only for ethical and legal reasons, but also to honor the client's rights as an individual.

There are also more subtle aspects to consider when writing about clients. Spaniol and Cattaneo (1994) emphasize how the use of words to describe clients or interact with them can easily become an ethical issue not only when talking with clients, but also when talking about them. They highlight the importance of non-judgmental language in descriptions of clients, noting that "many words and phrases commonly used in the mental health field imply judgment and too often become disparaging labels" (p. 269). They suggest a "people first language" (see Guidelines for Reporting and Writing about People with Disabilities, 1993) which delineates the use of vocabulary that supports an individual's integrity, emphasizing humanity over disability. Spaniol and Cattaneo underscore the need to be sensitive about language used not only in therapeutic interactions, but also in speaking and writing about clients.

Lastly, respect and sensitivity to both cultural and gender issues are important in scholarly writing. There are several good references in the resource list at the end of this chapter that describe the various problems and considerations in writing about multicultural and diverse populations.

## Professional Courtesy

An important ethical issue in scholarly writing and presentation is the concept of professional courtesy. Professional courtesy is the respect extended to colleagues, peers, teachers, and supervisors when using their original work in one's written publication or oral presentation. In publications, it may be in the form of citing the work of another in a reference list or it may be as simple as making an acknowledgment in a footnote of a person's contribution to the development of the work.

A very common instance where professional courtesy is extended is in the preface to a master's thesis or doctoral dissertation. It is a tradition for the author to note the people who contributed to development of the work, particularly teachers, supervisors, committee chairs and members, and mentors. This is a formal and effective way of acknowledging the information conveyed throughout the student's program of study as well as the time teachers, committee members, and others have put into the student's learning experience. In oral theses or dissertation presentations, the acknowledgment may be less formal, with the speaker briefly noting any individuals who inspired, provided professional communications, or helped to develop the ideas presented in the talk.

Unfortunately, lack of professional courtesy in publications and presentations in art therapy and other fields is a fairly common occurrence. Recently, I was stunned to see my exact words and original ideas from a graduate class I had taught at the local university in print in a magazine and credited to a former student, but with no reference to me included as the source for these concepts. It gave me pause to think how often I have heard art therapy educators observe that former students or supervisees used the original materials they have so carefully provided them in the classroom without acknowledging them as the source for these ideas. Part of the reason for this is that some students see their professors with consumers' eyes; they may believe what they receive in the classroom is something that they have purchased through tuition, and therefore becomes theirs to use in any manner. They are often naive in their understanding of what their mentors have put into their lectures, experientials, and course outlines in terms of time and research. Therefore, they may assume that they do not need to give reference to original material that is conveyed to them in an educational or supervisory setting. In the same vein, they may also usurp the ideas of fellow students, neglecting to acknowledge them as the source of inspiration, collegial advice, or communication.

Educators and supervisors also need to be wary of their inappropriate use of student work accomplished under their tutelage. It is not news that professors have used graduate students' work as their own in both publications and professional presentations. Therefore, the same courtesy must be considered when including the work of students within a paper or other scholarly presentation.

Professionals in our field are often guilty of not giving appropriate credit to others. Many papers are submitted to the journal with inadequate references to the original ideas developed by other art therapists. Some of this is due to lack of library research on the topic of the paper and certainly, the author has the choice to reference or not reference another author within the development of his/her topic. Unfortunately, at other times it is the result of professional jealousy or pettiness; by not referencing the ideas of others who have contributed information on a specific topic one somehow draws attention away from that contribution, giving more attention to one's own work. In either case, however, when ideas are presented that approximate the original work of another individual, then credit in some form must be given, either in the reference list (when cited within the text of the article or presentation) or in an acknowledgment (when a mentor, teacher, supervisor or colleague has significantly contributed to a paper/talk or advised the author/presenter).

The Ethics Committee of the American Art Therapy Association has developed a revised ethical code for art therapists, which addresses some of the issues of publication credit, professional courtesy, and respect for original ideas. The AATA ethics document brings to light another more serious dimension of scholarly writing: plagiarism. Plagiarism is an ethical transgression as well as a possible legal violation which involves stealing either the exact words or the ideas of another individual. The American Psychological Association (1992) defines plagiarism as follows:

> 6.22 Plagiarism. Psychologists do not present substantial portions or elements of another's work or data as their own, even if the other work or data source is cited occasionally. (APA, 1992)

The AATA ethics document does not directly address the concept on plagiarism per se. However, it does cover the related topic of professional courtesy with regard to publications and other printed materials. "Responsibility to the Profession", Section 7, states:

> 7.2 Art therapists shall attribute publication credit to those who have contributed to a publication in proportion to their contributions and in accordance with customary professional publication practices.

> 7.3 Art therapists who author books or other materials which are published or distributed shall appropriately cite persons to whom credit for original ideas is due. (AATA, 1995)

Others in the field of art therapy have examined this issue as well. In the document, *The Diagnostic Drawing Series Style Guide*, Mills (1994) suggests the following courtesy concerning citation of work derived from the DDS:

> When presenting work which derives from the DDS Archive, it is good form to acknowledge by name (verbally if presenting; in a footnote or author's note if publishing) the contributions of those who assisted by collecting the Series or by helping you on site. Extensive consultation with others about your work should also be acknowledged in this manner.

Professional courtesy in the field of art therapy is a subject that should be discussed with our students in their graduate training and with interns we supervise. It is also a practice that professionals should be cognizant of in their own writing and conference presentations. Aside from the obvious ethical aspects of the professional courtesy, there is an added benefit involving respect and affirmation of other's work. These are concepts that support art therapists in continuing to share their work either through publication or presentation, and affirm the value of one's original contributions to the field.

## Conclusion

This has been a very brief introduction to the area of scholarly writing and some of the ethical issues related to art therapy writing in general. The need to accurately, eloquently and substantially articulate our profession is at a critical point. In recent years, art therapists have been asked to demonstrate the value of our profession to a variety of sources. Some of these sources have included insurance care providers and health service regulating bodies. Still others have involved recognition and scrutiny from the federal government. As we continue to be recognized as a viable professional discipline, undoubtedly there will be other arenas in which we will have to publicly and credibly demonstrate our worth as a profession through our ability to write about art therapy both accurately and convincingly.

It is paramount that writing about art therapy theory, practice, and research be articulate and exacting, especially if art therapists want to demonstrate a unique knowledge base which is distinctly separate from other related disciplines. Needless to say, writing about research is particularly important, although art therapists have been squeamish to admit it and resistant to undertaking it. Scholarly writing often defines the profession of art therapy to others in related fields. Therefore, it is essential that authors consider the power that their written words have in shaping and defining art therapy as a discipline and endeavor to contribute material that is well-written, insightful, and substantive.

Note: Some of the material in this chapter has previously appeared in a different form in Art Therapy: Journal of the American Art Therapy Association (C. Malchiodi, ed.) in the following articles: Malchiodi, C.A. (1992). Writing for publication. *Art Therapy: Journal of the American Art Therapy Association* and Malchiodi, C.A. (1994). Professional courtesy. *Art Therapy: Journal of the American Art Therapy Association.*

## References

American Art Therapy Association. (1995). Ethical *standards for art therapists.* Mundelein, IL: Author.

Kramer, P.D. (1994). Private faces in public places: The ethics of writing about our clients. *Family Therapy Networker, 18,* 15-17.

Malchiodi, C.A. (1992). Writing for publication. *Art Therapy: Journal of the American Art Therapy Association, 9* (2), 62-64.

Malchiodi, C.A. (1994). Professional courtesy. *Art Therapy: Journal of the American Art Therapy Association, 11* (4), 242-243.

Mills, A. (1994). *The Diagnostic Drawing Series style guide.* Unpublished document available from the author.

Research and Training Center on Independent Living. (1993). *Guidelines for reporting and writing about people with disabilities. (3rd* ed.) Lawrence, KS: University of Kansas.

Rosal, M. (1989). Master's papers in art therapy: Narrative or research case studies? *The Arts in Psychotherapy, 16* (2), 71-75.

Spaniol, S., & Cattaneo, M. (1994). The power of language in the art therapeutic relationship. *Art Therapy: Journal of the American Art Therapy Association, 11* (4), 266-270.

**For additional information on authorship and style see:**

American Psychological Association. (1994). *Publication manual of the American Psychological Association* (4th ed.). Washington, DC: Author.

## Other Resources

American Association of University Presses. (1994). *Guidelines for bias-free usage.* New York: Author.

American Psychological Association. (1992). *PsycINFO Psychological Abstracts Information Services users reference manual.* Washington, DC: Author.

Boston, B. (1992). Portraying people with disabilities: Toward a new vocabulary. *The Editorial Eye, 15,* 1-3, 6-7.

Cone, J., & Foster, S. (1993). *Dissertations and theses from start to finish: Psychology and related fields.* Washington, DC: American Psychological Association.

Fine, M.A., & Kurdek, L. (1993). Reflections on determining authorship credit and authorship order on faculty-student collaborations. *American Psychologist, 48,* 1141-1147.

Gaw, A.C. (Ed.). (1993). *Culture, ethnicity, and mental illness*. Washington, DC: American Psychiatric Press.

Li, X., & Crane, N.B. (1993). *Electronic style: A guide to citing electronic information*. Westport, CT: Meckler.

Maggio, R. (1991). *The bias-free word finder: A dictionary of nondiscriminatory language*. Boston: Beacon Press.

Strunk, W., & White, E.B. (1979). *The elements of style* (3rd ed.). New York: Macmillan.

University of Chicago Press. (1993). *The Chicago manual of style*. (14th ed.) Chicago: Author.

Walker, A. (Ed.). (1994). *Thesaurus of psychological index terms* (7th ed.) . Washington, DC: American Psychological Association.

## Major Databases

This list is provided to familiarize authors with some of the available resources. These resources are available at most university libraries and on-line via Internet.

Index Medicus/MEDLINE
Child Development Abstracts
Dissertation Abstracts International
Exceptional Child Education Abstracts
PsycINFO/PsycLIT/Psychological Abstracts
ERIC (Education Resources Information Clearinghouse)
Current Content

## Other Resources for a Literature Review:

Because older art therapy literature is not included in current databases, these resources may be useful for some citations.

Gantt, L., & Schmal, M. (1974). *Art therapy: A bibliography*. Rockville, MD: National Institute of Mental Health. [annotated bibliography of art therapy literature from 1940-1973]

Hanes, K.M. (1982). *Art therapy and group work*. Westport, CT: Greenwood Press.

Moore, R. (1981). *Art therapy in mental health*. National Clearinghouse for Mental Health Information, Literature Survey Series #3, Rockville, MD: US Department of Health and Human Services.

# AN APA "CHEAT SHEET"

## Using Correct Citations:
One work by a single author:
1. Rubin (1984) compared the art expressions....
2. In a recent study of child art expressions (Rubin, 1984)....
3. In 1984, Rubin compared....

## Works by multiple authors:
Use an ampersand (&) in parenthetical material; use and in the text.
1. as Kagin and Lusebrink (1979) indicated....
2. as has been shown (Kagin & Lusebrink, 1979)....

## Examples of quotations of sources:
1. She stated, "The primary function of the art therapist is to create and maintain a working atmosphere" (Kramer, 1978, p. 276), but she did not clarify what kind of atmosphere.

2. Kramer (1978) noted that "the primary function of the art therapist is to create and maintain a working atmosphere" (p. 276).

3. For quotes of 40 or more words: Indent five to seven spaces from the left margin and do not single space. If the quote includes more than one paragraph, indent the first line of second and subsequent paragraphs five to seven spaces from the new margin.

Levick (1983) found that:

"During this period, the graphic productions of children seem to show the greatest differences, a conclusion derived from clinical experience. The growing child acquires new perceptions of known objects in the environment. Also, the acquisition of new perceptions and intellectual awareness of new objects and people in the environment also develops. These now become internalized." (p. 76)

## Alphabetize multiple authors in a list
(Adams, 1977; Downs & Jones, 1985; Zimmerman & Lennon, 1980)

## Cite all authors the first time the reference occurs if the work has more than one author and less than six.
Speight, Myers, Cox, & Highlen (1991) observed the need for redefinition of multicultural counseling....

Speight et al (1991) noted implications of redefinition include training, practice and research. [Subsequent citations include the first author's last name followed by et al.]

## Creating a Reference List:

Be sure to indent first line in each reference five spaces. Use lower case letters for book titles and journal article titles except for the first letter of the first word, first letter of proper nouns, and the first letter following a colon. (Note: Although APA style requires the first line to be indented, in most scholarly publications, the first line is not indented; rather the succeeding lines are indented. So use your own judgement when it comes to indentation!)

Book example:

Jones, P., & Smith, D. (1994). Capitalization using APA style: A guideline. Los Angeles: Generic Press.

Journal example:

Smith, D. (1994). The art of referencing. Journal of Libraries, 38 (2), 151-156.

The entire reference list is alphabetized by lead author.

## Journal article - one author:

Pavio, A. (1975). Perceptual comparisons through the mind's eye. Cognition, 3, 645-647.

[Author's name, year, title, title of journal, volume (use section number only if pages are not consecutively numbered through year), pages.]

## Book:

Barron, F. (1972). Artists in the making. New York: Seminar.

## Journal article - multiple authors:

Schaefer, C., Coyne, J. C., & Lazarus, R. S. (1982). The health-related functions of social support. Journal of Behavioral Medicine, 4, 381-406.

## Article or chapter in an edited book:

Silver, R. L., & Wortman, C. B. (1980). Coping with undesirable life events: In J. Garber & M.E.P. Seligman (Eds.), Human helplessness (pp. 245-270). New York: Academic Press.

## Other common errors:

—Do not use periods with capital letter abbreviations or acronyms, e.g. PhD, IQ, AATA; however, A.T.R. requires periods because it is trademarked as such.
—Use figures for numbers 10 and above unless the number begins the sentence.
—Use figures for numbers under 10 in certain instances
    If grouped for comparison with numbers 10 and above, e.g., 3 of 14 subjects.
    If the number precedes a specific measurement, e.g., 2 cm, 4 years, 1 weeks, 6 hours, 8 minutes.
    If you are referring to the subjects in your study, e.g., 2 subjects reported....
—Form the plural of years by adding "s" only, e.g., 1980s.

# APPENDIX A

## ART THERAPY SUPERVISION QUESTIONNAIRE

Dear Colleague:

We are collecting data on how art therapists supervise their students and interns. We would appreciate it if you would provide me with answers to the following questions. We will be happy to provide you with the results of this informal survey when it is completed.

Name: _____

Address:_____

_____

A.T.R. _____yes_____no

Other credentials_____

Primary Job Title:_____

How many individuals do you currently supervise? _____

Do you supervise ___undergraduate___graduate/Master's level
_____post-graduate

How many years have you been a supervisor?_____

Where/how did you learn to supervise?


Are you or have you ever been in a peer supervision group? If so, when and please provide a short description of group.


Where do you supervise? Check all that apply, but indicate most frequent site./type

_____on site where supervisee works (what type of facility?)

_____on site where you work (what type of facility?)

_____in school that supervisee attends (graduate or undergraduate?)

_____by phone

_____by mail

_____in home office

_____other (please describe)


In what capacity? Check all that apply

_____Individual

_____Group

What topics do you cover in supervisory sessions? Check all that apply and indicate the 3 most frequently discussed topics.

_____case material from clients

_____documentation/charting

_____ethics/ethical dilemmas

_____legal issues

_____professional credentials (registration, certification, licensure)

_____assessment

_____agency/institutional politics

_____art therapist identity

_____visual art

_____other (please describe)

Methods used in supervision. Check all that apply and indicate the most frequently used method.

_____verbal discussion

_____case presentation by supervisee(s)

_____art making by supervisee(s)

_____role play

_____videotape

_____other (please describe)

Overall, what do you feel are the most important issues to be addressed in the supervision of art therapy students or post-graduate art therapy interns?

What areas of art therapy supervision would you like to know more about?

# FORMS & CONTRACTS USED IN SUPERVISION

The following section of the Appendix provides sample forms and contracts used in supervision. Since supervisors are responsible for the actions of their supervisees, supervisors should maintain records of their supervisees' work, just as they do for their clients. Record-keeping may include, but is not limited to, any of the following: contractual agreements between the supervisor, supervisee and practicum/internship site; evaluations of the supervisee, practicum/internship site, and supervisor; time sheets; client progress notes; and release of client case materials, art expressions, and recordings.

Most graduate training programs have developed their own forms to record hours, evaluate practicum internship experiences, document client contact, and secure permission to use client materials. However, post-masters trainees and their supervisors are less likely to use formal documentation and evaluation forms in supervision; therefore, sample formats for recording hours, making evaluations of trainee progress, the practicum/internship site, and the supervisory experience, obtaining permission to use client case materials and art expressions are provided. The reader is advised to check any agency, state, or national regulations that may effect the format of documentation (e.g. agency/institutional policies and procedures, or state licensing and national certification boards).

Recording case material and writing progress notes are two other important components of practicums and internships. Forms and formats for this type of record keeping are provided in Chapter 11, Documentation and Case Presentation.

## APPENDIX B
# PRACTICUM LEARNING AGREEMENT

Trainee's name _____ Date _____

Address _____
_____ Phone _____

Practicum site _____

Address _____
_____ Phone _____

Supervisor's Name _____ Title _____

Supervisor's Degree, Credentials, & Licensure _____

Supervision: Individual (one hour)_____, Group (two hours)_____
     per:  direct service___  client contact___

Agency Director's Name_____

Learning Objectives for practicum experience _____
_____
_____
_____

Practicum Responsibilities & Schedule _____
_____
_____
_____

_____          _____
Student's signature                                              date

_____          _____
Supervisor's signature                                          date

## Practicum/Internship Weekly Time Sheet

Student:_____

Site:_____

Address:_____Phone:____/_____

Please list by hour the type of fieldwork experience, including preparation time, progress note writing, clinical conferences, work with individuals and groups, onsite supervision, and group supervision seminars. Use appropriate codes in your accounting.

Week of_____to_____

| MON | TUES | WED | THUR | FRI | SAT | SUN |
|-----|------|-----|------|-----|-----|-----|
|     |      |     |      |     |     |     |
|     |      |     |      |     |     |     |
|     |      |     |      |     |     |     |
|     |      |     |      |     |     |     |
|     |      |     |      |     |     |     |
|     |      |     |      |     |     |     |
|     |      |     |      |     |     |     |
|     |      |     |      |     |     |     |

___   ___   ___   ___   ___   ___   ___

Daily Totals

TOTAL HOURS FOR WEEK:_____ TOTAL HOURS TO DATE:_____

To the best of my knowledge, the information shown above is accurate:

_____     _____
On-site Supervisor          date     Supervisee              date

# CODES TO USE ON WEEKLY TIME SHEETS

**Client Contact Hours**

| | |
|---|---|
| Individual clients for therapy | IND |
| Couples | CPL |
| Families | FAM |
| Groups | GRP |
| Are present for a contact hours and clients do not show | NO SHOW |
| Teleconference with clients | TEL CONF |

**Supervision Hours**

| | |
|---|---|
| Attend Individual Supervision | IND SUPV |
| Attend Group Supervision | GRP SUPV |

**Other Hours**

| | |
|---|---|
| Preparation for client contact (getting materials ready, writing letters, brief telephone contacts, completing referral forms, brief discussions with on-site personnel or supervisors) | PREP |
| Writing clinical notes | CLN |
| Attending staff meetings | MTG |
| Outside related research and reading | RES |
| Attend workshops, lectures, conferences | WKSH LECT CONF |
| Program development/conduct inservice training | PDEV |

## APPENDIX C

# ART THERAPY SUPERVISION SEMINAR

# STATEMENT OF CONFIDENTIALITY

I am a member of [course number] which includes group discussion of clinical art therapy experiences that students have at placement sites. I understand that students in the course will be revealing information about themselves and their clients as part of the seminar and that confidentiality is necessary to establish trust and cohesion in the group and to respect clients' rights to privacy. In accordance with the ethics of confidentiality, what I see and hear within the seminar will be treated as privileged communication.


_____        _____

Signature                                    Date

# APPENDIX D

## SAMPLE CONTRACT FOR USING CLIENT ART**

Contract between _____and _____
                (art therapist's name)                   (artist/client's name)

I, _____ agree to allow _____
           (artist's name)                     (art therapist's name)

to use and/or display and/or photograph my artwork for the following purpose(s):

            _____Exhibition
            _____Publication in a professional journal
            _____Presentation at professional conferences
            _____Consultation with other mental health professionals
            _____Educational purposes

_____ I do    _____I do not    wish to remain anonymous

Signed _____ Date _____
                 (client's name)

\*\*\*\*\*\*\*\*\*\*\*\*\*\*\*\*\*\*\*\*\*\*\*\*\*\*\*\*\*\*\*\*\*\*\*\*\*\*\*\*\*\*\*\*\*\*\*\*

I, _____(art therapist's name)_____, agree to the following conditions in connection with my use of artwork by_____(client's name)_____ :

I agree to safeguard your artwork to the best of my ability and to notify you immediately of any loss or damage while your art is in my possession.

I agree to provide an appropriate format for presentation if I exhibit your artwork, and to bear other costs related to the exhibition.

I agree to return your artwork immediately if you decide to withdraw your consent. I also agree to safeguard your confidentiality.

Signed: _____ Date_____
              (art therapist's name)

**This was originally published in the *American Journal of Art Therapy, 32* (3), 1994, with the title "Confidentiality Reexamined: Negotiating Use of Art by Clients," by Susan Spaniol, EdD, A.T.R., LMHC, and is reprinted here with permission of Vermont College of Norwich University.

# APPENDIX E

## CONSENT TO USE AND DISPLAY

## ART THERAPY WORK PRODUCTS**

I, _____, give permission to

_____, to use and/or
display art work created by me in a professional setting for the purpose of
supervision or education on the therapeutic use of art therapy. It is my
understanding that my name will not be revealed in any presentation or display
of my art work.

This consent to disclose may be revoked by me at any time except to the
extent that action has been taken in reliance thereon.


Patient/Client_____ Date_____

Witness_____ Date_____


**This was originally published in the *American Journal of Art Therapy, 32*
(3), 1994, with the title "Confidentiality Reexamined: Negotiating Use of Art by
Clients," by Susan Spaniol, EdD, A.T.R., LMHC, and is reprinted here with
permission of Vermont College of Norwich University.

## APPENDIX F

# PERMISSION TO AUDIOTAPE OR VIDEOTAPE

I give my permission to _____

to record on audiotape/videotape my participation in _____

_____

I have been informed that the recording will be kept strictly confidential and the recording is solely for the purpose of clinical treatment, educational purposes, and/or supervision. The interviewer will retain the audiotape/videotape in order to ensure confidentiality and access to them will be limited to the above mentioned purposes.

Client_____ Date _____

Witness _____ Date _____

## APPENDIX G

# FINAL EVALUATION OF PRACTICUM/INTERNSHIP
# EXPERIENCE

Student:_____
Practicum/Internship site:_____
Supervisor:_____

Total number of hours completed by the student at this site:_____
Total number of direct client contact hours completed by the student at this
site:_____
Total number of individual supervision hours the student received:_____

### 1. Overall Clinical Skills
a) Demonstrates an understanding of why the client sought treatment
                          1       2       3       4       5
b) Demonstrates understanding of how the client's history relates to the
presenting problems          1       2       3       4       5
c) Demonstrates understanding of client's motivation for treatment
                          1       2       3       4       5
d) Demonstrates understanding of the client's resistance to treatment
                          1       2       3       4       5
e) Demonstrates understanding of the client-therapist relationship
and how this may relate to the client's presenting problem, history and
interactional style          1       2       3       4       5
f) Demonstrates understanding of theory as it is applied to therapeutic process
                          1       2       3       4       5
g) Demonstrates ability to confront
                          1       2       3       4       5
h) Demonstrates ability to support and set limits
                          1       2       3       4       5
i) Able to terminate effectively
                          1       2       3       4       5
j) Recognizes and deals with transference
                          1       2       3       4       5
k) Recognizes and deals with countertransference
                          1       2       3       4       5
Comments:_____

## 2. Treatment Goals
a) Defines both client and therapist treatment goals

                                      1      2      3      4      5

b) Sets short-term, intermediate and long-term goals

    1      2      3      4      5

c) Translates goals into observable and/or measurable outcomes

    1      2      3      4      5

d) Is able to change goals over the course of treatment as needed

    1      2      3      4      5

Comments:_____

## 3. Interventional Skills
a) Has clear rationale for providing interventions

    1      2      3      4      5

b) Appropriately paces interventions to client's abilities and current status

    1      2      3      4      5

c) Chooses interventions with a clear understanding of time restrictions, frequency of sessions, etc.    1      2      3      4      5

d) Chooses interventions with a clear understanding of materials and media variables    1      2      3      4      5

e) Considers alternative interventions

    1      2      3      4      5

f) Understands limitations and possible negative consequences of interventions used    1      2      3      4      5

Comments:_____

## 4. Treatment of Art Expressions
a) Obtains appropriate permission for display and presentation

    1      2      3      4      5

b) Treats art expressions with care and ethical responsibility

    1      2      3      4      5

c) Follows procedures for confidentiality

    1      2      3      4      5

d) Discusses art expressions with respect for client and the art expression

    1      2      3      4      5

e) Demonstrates understanding of theory with regard to the content of art expressions    1      2      3      4      5

Comments:_____

_____

### 5. Progress Evaluation
a) Has clear criteria for the evaluation of progress

                 1     2     3     4     5

b) Checks progress with client

                 1     2     3     4     5

c) Checks progress with colleagues/supervisors

                 1     2     3     4     5

d) Revises goals and interventions as necessary

                 1     2     3     4     5

e) Can support a link between interventions and the outcome of treatment

                 1     2     3     4     5

Comments:_____

_____

### 6. Professionalism
a) Uses effective and ethical case management skills

                 1     2     3     4     5

b) Is aware of potential ethical and legal issues relevant to case

                 1     2     3     4     5

c) Demonstrates ethical and responsible involvement with colleagues and agency          1     2     3     4     5

d) Maintains overall professional appearance and behavior

                 1     2     3     4     5

e) Demonstrates knowledge of laws and regulations affecting therapy

                 1     2     3     4     5

Comments:_____

_____

### 7. Use of Supervision:
a) Prepares for supervision

                 1     2     3     4     5

b) Actively participates in evaluation and self-critique

                 1     2     3     4     5

c) Open to learning from supervisor

                 1     2     3     4     5

d) Able to share feelings about the clients

                 1     2     3     4     5

e) Questions and challenges the supervisor

           1      2      3      4      5

f) Aware of own dynamics  with supervisor

           1      2      3      4      5

Comments:_____

_____


Any additional comments:_____

_____

_____

_____

## APPENDIX H

# PRACTICUM SITE EVALUATION

(to be completed by trainee at completion of practicum)

Student:_____ Date:_____

Site:_____

Address:_____

_____

Phone:_____/_____

Supervisor:_____

### Description of Practicum Site

Hours per week spent in placement:_____

Types of case assignments (individual, group, and/or family; co-therapy, adjunctive, and/or primary):_____

_____

_____

Please describe client population(s):_____

_____

_____

Staff meetings or seminars regularly attended:_____

_____

Positive features of the practicum site:_____

_____

_____

Negative features of the practicum site:_____

_____

_____

Staff acceptance of art therapy:_____

_____

_____

# APPENDIX I

## STUDENT EVALUATION OF SUPERVISOR

**I. General**
Was supervision conducted on a regular basis/schedule?

Was supervision timely, in a appropriate space, and adequate in length?

If your supervisor did not work at the practicum site where you were placed, was there sufficient communication between your supervisor and the agency?

Did you receive adequate educational support from your supervisor?

What methods did your supervisor use to enrich the supervisory sessions?

**II. Case Management**
Did your supervisor discuss
Treatment planning?

The clients' art process and products?

Interventions to accomplish established goals?

Your feelings regarding clients (e.g. transference/countertransference)?

Staff interaction and policies of the agency?

**III. Please make any additional comments about the supervisory experience.**

## APPENDIX J

# ETHICAL STANDARDS FOR ART THERAPISTS

(includes Guidelines for Independent Practitioners)

The Board of Directors of the American Art Therapy Association (AATA) hereby promulgate, pursuant to Article 8, Sections 1, 2, and 3 of the Association Bylaws, a Revised Code of Ethical Standards for Art Therapists. Members of AATA abide by these standards and by applicable state laws and regulations governing the conduct of art therapists and any additional license or certification which the art therapist holds.

## STANDARDS

## 1.0 RESPONSIBILITY TO PATIENTS

Art therapists shall advance the welfare of all patients, respect the rights of those persons seeking their assistance, and make reasonable efforts to ensure that their services are used appropriately.

1.1 Art therapists shall not discriminate against or refuse professional service to anyone on the basis of race, gender, religion, national origin, age, sexual orientation or disability.

1.2 At the outset of the patient-therapist relationship, art therapists shall discuss and explain to patients the rights, roles, expectations, and limitations of the art therapy process.

1.3 Where the patient is a minor, any and all disclosure or consent required hereunder shall be made to or obtained from the parent or legal guardian of the minor patient, except where otherwise provided by state law. Care shall be taken to preserve confidentiality with the minor patient and to refrain from disclosure of information to the parent or guardian which might adversely affect the treatment of the patient.

1.4 Art therapists shall respect the rights of patients to make decisions and shall assist them in understanding the consequences of these decisions. Art therapists advise their patients that decisions on the status of therapeutic relationships is the responsibility of the patient. It is the professional responsibility of the art therapist to avoid ambiguity in the therapeutic relationship and to ensure clarity of roles at all times

1.5 Art therapists shall not engage in dual relationships with patients. Art therapists shall recognize their influential position with respect to patients, and they shall not exploit the trust and dependency of persons. A dual relationship occurs when a therapist and patient engage in separate and distinct relationship(s) or when an instructor or supervisor acts as a therapist to a student or a supervisee either simultaneously with the therapeutic relationship, or less than two (2) years following termination of the therapeutic relationship. Some examples of dual relationships are borrowing money from the patient, hiring the patient, engaging in a business venture with the patient, engaging in a close personal relationship with the patient, or engaging in sexual intimacy with a patient.

1.6 Art therapists shall take appropriate professional precautions to ensure that their judgment is not impaired, that no exploitation occurs, and that all conduct is undertaken solely in the patient's best interest.

1.7 Art therapists shall not use their professional relationships with patients to further their own interests.

1.8 Art therapists shall continue a therapeutic relationship only so long as it is reasonably clear that the patient is benefiting from the relationship. It is unethical to maintain a professional or therapeutic relationship for the sole purpose of financial remuneration to the art therapist or when it becomes reasonably clear that the relationship or therapy is not in the best interest of the patient.

1.9 Art therapists shall not engage in therapy practices or procedures that are beyond their scope of practice, experience, training and education. Art therapists shall assist persons in obtaining other therapeutic services if the therapist is unable or unwilling, for appropriate reasons, to provide professional help, or where the problem or treatment indicated is beyond the scope of practice of the art therapist.

1.10 Art therapists shall not abandon or neglect patients in treatment. If the art therapist is unable to continue to provide professional help, the art therapist will assist the patient in making reasonable, alternative arrangements for continuation of treatment.

## 2.0 CONFIDENTIALITY

Art therapists shall respect and protect confidential information obtained from patients in conversation and/or through artistic expression.

2.1 Art therapists shall treat patients in an environment that protects privacy and confidentiality.

2.2 Art therapists shall protect the confidentiality of the patient therapist relationship in all matters.

2.3 Art therapists shall not disclose confidential information without patient's explicit written consent unless there is reason to believe that the client or others are in immediate, severe danger to health or life. Any such disclosure shall be consistent with state and federal laws that pertain to welfare of the patient, family, and the general public.

2.4 In the event that an art therapist believes it is in the interest of the patient to disclose confidential information, he/she shall seek and obtain written authorization from the patient or patient's guardian(s), before making any disclosures.

2.5 Art therapists shall disclose confidential information when mandated by law in a civil, criminal, or disciplinary action arising from the art therapy. In these cases patient confidences may only be disclosed as reasonably necessary in the course of that action.

2.6 Art therapists shall maintain patient treatment records for a reasonable amount of time consistent with state regulations and sound clinical practice, but not less than seven years from completion of treatment or termination of the therapeutic relationship. Records are stored or disposed of in ways that maintain confidentiality.

## 3.0 PUBLIC USE AND REPRODUCTION OF PATIENT ART EXPRESSION AND THERAPY SESSIONS

Art therapists shall not make or permit any public use or reproduction of the patients' art therapy sessions, including dialogue and art expression, without express written consent of the patient.

3.1 Art therapists shall obtain written informed consent from the patient or, where applicable, a legal guardian before photographing patients' art expressions, video taping, audio recording, or otherwise duplicating, or permitting third party observation of art therapy sessions.

3.2 Art therapists shall only use clinical materials in teaching, writing, and public presentations if a written authorization has been previously obtained from the patients. Appropriate steps shall be taken to protect patient identity and disguise any part of the art expression or video tape which reveals patient identity.

3.3 Art therapists shall obtain written, informed consent from the patient before displaying patient's art in galleries, in mental health facilities, schools, or other public places.

3.4 Art therapists may display patient art expression in an appropriate and dignified manner only when authorized by the patient in writing.

## 4.0 PROFESSIONAL COMPETENCE AND INTEGRITY

Art therapists shall maintain high standards of professional competence and integrity.

4.1 Art therapists shall keep informed and up-dated with regard to developments in their field through educational activities and clinical experiences. They shall also remain informed of developments in other fields in which they are licensed or certified, or which relate to their practice.

4.2 Art therapists shall diagnose, treat, or advise on problems only in those cases in which they are competent as determined by their education, training and experience.

4.3 Art therapists shall not provide professional services to a person receiving treatment or therapy from another professional, except by agreement with such other professional, or after termination of the patient's relationship with the other professional.

4.4 Art therapists, because of their potential to influence and alter the lives of others, shall exercise special care when making public their professional recommendations and opinions through testimony or other public statements.

4.5 Art therapists shall seek appropriate professional consultation or assistance for their personal problems or conflicts that may impair or affect work performance or clinical judgment.

4.6 Art therapists shall not engage in any relationship with patients, students, interns, trainees, supervises, employees or colleagues that is exploitive by its nature or effect.

4.7 Art therapists shall not distort or misuse their clinical and research findings.

4.8 Art therapists shall be in violation of this Code and subject to termination of membership or other appropriate actions if they:  a) are convicted of a crime substantially related to or impacting upon their professional qualifications or functions; b) are expelled from or disciplined by other professional organizations; c) have their license(s) or certificate(s) suspended or revoked or are otherwise disciplined by regulatory bodies; d) continue to practice when impaired due to medical or mental causes or the abuse of alcohol or other substances that would prohibit good judgment; or e) fail to cooperate with the American Art Therapy Association or the Ethics Committee, or any body found or convened by them at any point from the inception of an ethical complaint through the completion of all proceedings regarding that complaint.

## 5.0 RESPONSIBILITY TO STUDENTS AND SUPERVISEES

Art therapists shall instruct their students using accurate, current, and scholarly information and will, at all times, foster the professional growth of students and advisees.

5.1 Art therapists as teachers, supervisors and researchers shall maintain high standards of scholarship and present accurate information.

5.2 Art therapists shall be aware of their influential position with respect to students and supervisees and they shall avoid exploiting the trust and dependency of such persons.  Art therapists, therefore, shall not engage in a therapeutic relationship with their students or supervisees.  Provision of therapy to students or supervisees is unethical.

5.3 Art therapists shall not permit students, employees or supervisees to perform or to hold themselves out as competent to perform professional services beyond their education, training, level of experience or competence.

5.4 Art therapists who act as supervisors shall be responsible for maintaining the quality of their supervision skills and obtain consultation or supervision for their work as supervisors whenever appropriate.

## 6.0 RESPONSIBILITY TO RESEARCH PARTICIPANTS

Researchers shall respect the dignity and protect the welfare of participants in research.

6.1 Researchers shall be aware of federal and state laws and regulations and professional standards governing the conduct of research.

6.2 Researchers shall be responsible for making careful examinations of ethical acceptability in planning studies. To the extent that services to research participants may be compromised by participation in research, investigators shall seek the ethical advice of qualified professionals not directly involved in the investigation and shall observe safeguards to protect the rights of research participants.

6.3 Researchers requesting participants' involvement in research shall inform them of all aspects of the research that might reasonably be expected to influence willingness to participate. Investigators shall be especially sensitive to the possibility of diminished consent when participants are also receiving clinical services, have impairments which limit understanding and/or communication, or when participants are children.

6.4 Researchers shall respect participants freedom to decline participation in or to withdraw from a research study at any time. This obligation requires special thought and consideration when investigators or other members of the research team are in positions of authority or influence over participants. Art therapists, therefore, shall avoid dual relationships with research participants.

6.5 Information obtained about a research participant during the course of an investigation shall be confidential unless there is an authorization previously obtained in writing. When there is a risk that others, including family members, may obtain access to such information, this risk, together with the plan for protecting confidentiality, is to be explained as part of the procedure for obtaining informed consent.

## 7.0 RESPONSIBILITY TO THE PROFESSION

Art therapists shall respect the rights and responsibilities of professional colleagues and participate in activities which advance the goals of art therapy.

7.1 Art therapists shall adhere to the standards of the profession when acting as members or employees of organizations.

7.2 Art therapists shall attribute publication credit to those who have contributed to a publication in proportion to their contributions and in accordance with customary professional publication practices.

7.3 Art therapists who author books or other materials which are published or distributed shall appropriately cite persons to whom credit for original ideas is due.

7.4 Art therapists who author books or other materials published or distributed by an organization shall take reasonable precautions to ensure that the organization promotes and advertises the materials accurately and factually.

7.5 Art therapists shall recognize a responsibility to participate in activities that contribute to a better community and society, including devoting a portion of their professional activity to services for which there is little or no financial return.

7.6 Art therapists shall assist and be involved in developing laws and regulations pertaining to the field of art therapy which serve the public interest and with changing such laws and regulations that are not in the public interest.

7.7 Art therapists shall cooperate with the Ethics Committee of the American Art Therapy Association, Inc. and truthfully represent and disclose facts to the Ethics Committee when requested or when necessary to preserve the integrity of the art therapy profession.

7.8 Art therapists shall endeavor to prevent distortion, misuse or suppression of art therapy findings by any institution or agency of which they are employees.

## 8.0 FINANCIAL ARRANGEMENTS

Art therapists shall make financial arrangements with patients, third party payers and supervisees that are understandable and conform to accepted professional practices.

8.1 Art therapists shall not offer or accept payment for referrals.

8.2 Art therapists shall not exploit their patient financially.

8.3 Art therapists shall disclose their fees at the commencement of services and give reasonable notice of any changes in fees.

8.4 Art therapists shall represent facts truthfully to patients, third party payers and supervisees regarding services rendered and the charges therefore.

## 9.0 ADVERTISING

Art therapists shall engage in appropriate informational activities to enable lay persons to choose professional services on an informed basis.

9.1 Art therapists shall accurately represent their competence, education, training and experience relevant to their professional practice.

9.2 Art therapists shall assure that all advertisements and publications, whether in directories, announcement cards, newspapers, or on radio or television are formulated to accurately convey in a dignified and professional manner, information that is necessary for the public to make an informed, knowledgeable decision.

9.3 Art therapists shall not use a name which is likely to mislead the public concerning the identity, responsibility, source and status of those under whom they are practicing, and shall not hold themselves out as being partners or associates of a firm if they are not.

9.4 Art therapists shall not use any professional identification (such as a business card, office sign, letterhead, or telephone or association directory listing) if it includes a statement or claim that is false, fraudulent, misleading or deceptive. A statement is false, fraudulent, misleading or deceptive if it: a) fails to state any material fact necessary to keep the statement from being misleading; b) is intended to, or likely to, create an unjustified expectation or, c) contains a material misrepresentation of fact.

9.5 Art therapists shall correct, whenever possible, false, misleading, or inaccurate information and representations made by others concerning the therapist's qualifications, services or products.

9.6 Art therapists shall make certain that the qualifications of persons in their employ are represented in a manner that is not false, misleading or deceptive.

9.7 Art therapists may represent themselves as specializing within a limited area of art therapy only if they have the education, training and experience which meet recognized professional standards to practice in that specialty area.

9.8 AATA credentialed professional, professional, associate and other members in good standing may identify such membership in AATA in public information or advertising materials, but they must clearly and accurately represent the membership category to which they belong.

9.9 Art therapists shall not use the A.T.R. and/or A.T.R.-BC following their name unless they are officially notified in writing by the Art Therapy Credential Board, Inc. that they have successfully completed all applicable registration or certification procedures. Art therapists may not use the initials AATA following their name like an academic degree.

9.10 Art therapists may not use the AATA initials or logo without receiving written permission from the Association.

## 10.0 INDEPENDENT PRACTITIONER

DEFINITION: The Independent Practitioner of Art Therapy is a Credentialed Professional Member of the American Art Therapy Association, Inc. (AATA) who is practicing art therapy independently and who is responsible for the delivery of services to patients where the patient pays the clinician directly or through insurance for art therapy service rendered.

**GUIDELINES:**
10.1 Independent practitioners of art therapy shall maintain Registration with Art Therapy Credentials Board, Inc. (ATCB) and shall have in addition to their Registration at least two full years of full-time practice or 3,000 hours of paid clinical art therapy experience.
10.2 Independent practitioners of art therapy shall obtain qualified medical or psychological consultation for cases in which such evaluation and/or administration of medication is required. Art therapists shall not provide services other than art therapy unless licensed to provide such other services.
10.3 Independent practitioners of art therapy must conform to relevant federal, state and local government statutes which pertain to the provision of independent mental health practice. (Laws vary from state to state.) It is the sole responsibility of the independent practitioner to conform to these laws.
10.4 Independent practitioners of art therapy shall confine their practice within the limits of their training. The art therapist shall neither claim nor imply professional qualifications exceeding those actually earned and received by then. The therapist is responsible for avoiding and/or correcting any misrepresentation of these qualifications. Art therapists must adhere to state laws regarding independent practice and licensure, as applicable.

**ENVIRONMENT**
11.0 Independent practitioners of art therapy must provide a safe, functional environment in which to offer art therapy services. This includes:
  a. proper ventilation.
  b. adequate lighting.
  c. access to water supply.
  d. knowledge of hazards or toxicity of art materials and the effort needed to safeguard the health of clients.
  e. storage space for art projects and secured areas for any hazardous materials.
  f. monitored use of sharps.
  g. allowance for privacy and confidentiality.
  h. compliance with any other health and safety requirements according to state and federal agencies which regulate comparable businesses.

**REFERRAL AND ACCEPTANCE**
12.0 Independent practitioners of art therapy, upon acceptance of a patient, shall specify to patients their fee structure, payment schedule, session scheduling arrangements, and information pertaining to the limits of confidentiality and the duty to report.

**TREATMENT PLANNING**
13.0 Independent practitioners of art therapy shall design treatment plans:

a. to assist the patient in attaining maintenance of the maximum level of functioning and quality of life appropriate for each individual.

b. in compliance with federal state, and local regulations and any licensure requirements governing the provision of art therapy services in the state.

c. that delineate the type, frequency and duration of art therapy involvement.

d. that contain goals that reflect the patient's current needs and strengths. When possible, these goals are formulated with the patient's understanding and permission.

e. provide for timely review, modification and revision.

# DOCUMENTATION

14.0 Independent practitioners of art therapy shall document activity with patients so that the most recent art therapy progress notes reflect the following:

a. current level of functioning.

b. current goals of treatment plan.

c. verbal content of art therapy sessions relevant to client behavior and goals.

d. graphic images relevant to client behavior and goals

e. changes in affect, thought process, and behavior.

f. no change in affect, thought process, and behavior.

g. suicidal or homicidal intent or ideation.

14.1 Upon termination of the therapeutic relationship, independent practitioners of art therapy shall write a discharge/transfer summary that includes the patient's response to treatment and future treatment recommendations.

# TERMINATION OF SERVICES

15.0 Independent practitioners of art therapy shall terminate art therapy when the patient has attained stated goals and objectives or fails to benefit from art therapy services.

15.1 Independent practitioners of art therapy shall communicate the termination of art therapy services to the patient.

---

*Certain portions of these Ethical Standards are adapted from the American Association for Marriage and Family Therapy Code of Ethics (1991) with their permission.*

# APPENDIX K

## AMERICAN ART THERAPY ASSOCIATION

# General Standards of Practice for Art

# Therapists

## Preamble

Clinical standards of practice and principles of conduct have evolved in the field of art therapy since its organization in 1969. These principles have guided the relationships of the members of the profession to their clients, to each other, and to the community of which they are members. Some of these guidelines have been derived from the American Art Therapy Association Code of Ethics. A sign of maturity of our profession is the publication of these guiding principles and practices. This serves the best interest of the profession, its users, and the community at large. Because the practice of art therapy is evolving, guidelines for practice will require the addition of standards, periodic review, and revision.

These guidelines are offered as a set of goals to encourage the art therapist to strive to continually improve the quality of practice and service. Providers of art therapy services have the same responsibility to uphold these general guidelines as they would the corresponding Code of Ethics.

Because these general guidelines are less specific in nature, they are intended for use by all providers of art therapy services. They will be supplemented by specific guidelines for each specialty service developed.

These guidelines are intended to improve the quality, effectiveness, and accessibility of art therapy services.

## INTRODUCTION

The American Art Therapy Association Standards of Practice provide guidelines for Art Therapists and those using art therapy services. These standards were developed by the Clinical Committee of the American Art Therapy Association. Registered art therapists are expected to follow these guidelines.

Glossary of terms
- Assessment -The use of any combination of verbal, written, and art tasks chosen by the professional art therapist to assess the individual's level of functioning, problem areas, strengths, and treatment objectives.
- Providers of Art Therapy Services
  A. Professional Art Therapist: Master's degree or (equivalent) from an accredited program in Art Therapy and/or Registered Art Therapist (A.T.R.).
- Art Therapist Service Unit:
  This is a functional unit in which Art Therapy services are provided:
  A. An art therapy service unit is a unit that provides predominantly art therapy services and is composed of one or more professional art therapists and support staff.
  B. An art therapy service may operate as a functional or geographic component of a larger governmental, educational, correctional, health training, industrial, or commercial organizational unit, or as an independent professional service unit.
  C. An art therapy service may take the form of one or more therapists providing professional services in a multidisciplinary setting.
  D. An art therapy service unit may also be an individual or group of individuals in a private practice or consultation services.
- Users:
  Clients include the following :
  A. Direct users or recipients of art therapy services.
  B. Public and private institutions, facilities, or organizations receiving art therapy services.
- Sanctioners:
  Sanctioners include the following:
  A. Direct users or recipients of art therapy services.
  B. Public and private institutions, facilities, or organizations receiving art therapy services.
  C. Any other individual, group, organization, or governing body having legitimate interaction with an art therapist functioning in a professional capacity.

## GENERAL GUIDELINES I: Providers
1.1 Each art therapy unit offering art therapy services has available at least one professional art therapist and as many more professional art therapists as are necessary to assure the quality of services offered.

1.2 of art therapy services who do not meet the requirements for professional art therapist are supervised, directed, and evaluated by a professional art therapist to the extent required by the task assigned. Tasks assigned to these providers are in keeping with their demonstrated levels and areas of competence.

1.3.1 Wherever an art therapist service unit exists, a professional art therapist is responsible for planning, directing, and evaluating the provision of these services including any revisions required.

1.4 When the work setting is a large organization, the professional art therapist seeks, when appropriate, to impact the goals of the organization by participating in the planning and development of overall operations.

1.5 All providers of art therapy services attempt to maintain current knowledge of professional developments that are directly related to the services they render. This should include active planning of continuing education programs to maximize quality of services rendered to art therapy users. Knowledge in areas relating to special populations (such as ethnic or other minorities) that may compose a part of their practice is particularly important.

1.6 Art therapists are encouraged to develop and evaluate innovative theories, to participate in clinical research to enhance the scientific basis of the field, and to disseminate their results to others.

1.7 Providers of art therapy services avoid any action that will violate or diminish the legal and civil rights of users or of others who may be affected by their actions.

1.8 Providers of art therapy services are familiar with and abide by the American Art Therapy Association, Inc. rules, regulations, and Code of Ethics.

1.9 Providers of art therapy services will seek to conform to relevant federal, state, and local government statutes.

1.10 Providers of art therapy services do not use privileged information received in the course of their work for competitive advantage.

## GENERAL GUIDELINES II: Programs

2.0.0 Each art therapy service unit is guided by a set of procedural guidelines for the delivery of art therapy services.

2.0.1 A written description of roles, objectives, and scope of services is developed by art therapy service units as well as by other units that are a component of an organization. The written description is reviewed annually and is made available to the staff of the unit and to clients upon request.

*Standard I: Referral and Acceptance*

The following criteria is considered when accepting art therapy clients:

2.1 A client is a candidate for art therapy unless she/he is inappropriate for this specific treatment modality.

2.2 A client may be referred for an initial art therapy assessment by: a professional therapist, others, members of other disciplines, self

2.3 The final decision to accept a client for art therapy services, either direct or consultative, is made by a professional art therapist.

2.4 The professional art therapist clarifies early on to users and sanctioners the exact fee structure or financial arrangements and payment schedule when providing service for a fee.

2.5 A client is assessed by a professional art therapist or an art therapist under supervision prior to the delivery of art therapy services

*Standard II: Assessment*

2.2.0 The art therapy assessment reflects the psychosocial, educational, developmental, and behavioral functioning as related to the clients needs and shall focus on major conflicts, defenses, strengths, and art training.

2.2.1 The assessment includes a combination of verbal, written or art tasks deemed most appropriate by the art therapist to ascertain individual client goals, treatment objectives, and recommendations for further treatment.

2.2.2 The assessment recognizes variability of performance resulting from medications, psychosocial conditions, art training, cultural background, and current health status.

2.2.3 All interpretation of assessment methods shall be based on current literature and research of other art therapists as well as literature and research in related fields.

2.2.4 The results, conclusions, and implications of the art therapy assessment shall become the basis for the client's art therapy program and shall be communicated to others concerned with provision of services to the client and through documentation in the client's record. In understandable language and in accordance with the art therapist's clinical judgement, the results are communicated to the client.

2.2.5 When assessment indicates the client's need for other services, the professional art therapist shall communicate this to the treatment team or other clinicians involved in the treatment. Information regarding additional human services, such as specialized art therapy services, legal aid societies, social services, employment agencies, health resources, and educational and recreational facilities will be supplied as deemed appropriate since art therapy is one form of treatment in a wide spectrum of therapies available.

*Standard III: Program Planning*
From the evaluation process, the professional art therapist develops an individual treatment plan. The art therapy evaluation goals and recommendations are reviewed and, when possible, followed up in meetings with the treatment team and/or other treaters. The art therapy treatment plan:
2.3.0 Is designed to assist the client attain and maintain the maximum level of functioning and quality of life.
2.3.1 Is in compliance with federal, state, and facilities regulations.
2.3.2 Delineates the type, frequency and duration of art therapy involvement.
2.3.3 Contains goals and measurable objectives that reflect the client's needs and strengths.
2.3.4 Provides for timely assessment and appropriate modifications of treatment plans.
2.3.5 Is consistent with the following according to the best professional judgement of the art therapist:
  a. the program plans of other disciplines.
  b. established principles of growth and development.

*Standard IV: Implementation*
The professional art therapist delivers services according to the individualized treatment plan:
2.4.0 Strives for the highest level and quality of art involvement consistent with the functioning level of the client.
2.4.1 Offers appropriate art materials, techniques and exercises relating to client's needs and goals.
2.4.2 Uses methodology that is consistent with standard health and safety procedures.
2.4.3 Records and evaluates the client's response to determine the progress.

*Standard V: Documentation*
2.5.0 The frequency of documentation shall be established so that the most recent art therapy progress notes reflect accurately:
  a. Current level of functioning
  b. Current goals and treatment plan
  c. Content and graphic features related to problem
  d. New changes in affect, thought process, and behavior
2.5.1 An art therapy discharge/transfer summary or progress note shall be written including response to treatment and recommendations.
2.5.2 Each art therapy service unit follows an established policy for the

retention and disposition of records.

2.5.3 The art therpist will closely follow existing institution or professional guidelines for confidentiality regarding records and art work.

*Standard VI: Termination of Services*

The professional art therapist shall terminate art therapy when the client has attained stated goals and objectives, fails to benefit from services, or is discharged/transferred.

2.6.0 The professional art therapist shall communicate the termination of art therapy services. The termination plan will be consistent with the individualized art therapy treatment plan.

2.6.1 At the time of termination, the professional art therapist shall schedule sessions to review progress and when feasible return artwork to client.

2.6.2 Termination report shall include record of client attendance and progress, any unresolved conficts, and further recommendations.

## GENERAL GUIDELINE III: Accountability

3.0 In the public interest, the professional art therapist may wish to provide some services to individuals or organizations on a sliding fee scale for little or no financial return.

3.1 The promotion of human welfare is the primary principle guiding the professional activities of all members of the art therapy service.

3.2 The art therapist provides services in a non-discriminatory and non-exploitive manner and follows professional and ethical standards devised by the American Art Therapy Association.

3.3 The client will be informed prior to changes in the delivery of treatment.

## GUIDELINE IV: Environment

4.0 The professional art therapist is responsible for the safety of the environment by implementing rules and guidelines for safety.

4.0.1 The environment should include but is not limited to:

a. proper ventilation

b. adequate lighting

c. access to water supply

d. storage space for art projects and secured areas for any hazardous materials

e. monitored use of sharps

f. the space should ensure privacy and confidentiality

g. the space should meet other health and safety requirements from the facility, state, and federal agencies

# APPENDIX L

# COUNSELING & THERAPIST PRACTICE ACT, SECTION 16

The following rules concerning supervision were established by the New Mexico Counseling and Therapy Practice Board, Regulation and Licensing Department during 1994; because this legislation establishes rules for licensure and supervision of art therapists, it is an important resource for understanding how supervision is defined by law:

16.1 Approved Supervisor Definitions

A. Administrative supervision means those supervisory activities which increase the efficiency of the delivery of counseling services.

B. Clinical supervision means the supportive and educative activities of the supervisor designed to improve the application of counseling theory and technique directly to clients. Clinical supervision is the only supervision acceptable for licensure.

C. Applied counseling settings means public or private organizations of counselors and therapists such as community mental health counselors, hospitals, schools, and group or individual private practice settings.

D. Supervisees means licensees who are working with clients in an applied counseling setting.

E. Supervisors means counselors and therapists or other approved supervisors as defined in Rule 2.4 who within applied counseling settings oversee the professional clinical work of registered mental health counselors or licensees.

16.2 Supervisee's Welfare and Rights

A. Supervisors shall instruct supervisees to notify clients that they are being supervised and that observation and/or recordings of the session may be reviewed by the supervisor.

B. Supervisors who are licensed counselors and therapists and are conducting supervision to aid a supervisees to become licensed shall instruct the supervisee not to communicate or in anyway convey to the supervisee's clients or to other parties that the supervisee is himself/herself licensed.

C. Supervisors shall instruct supervisees of client's rights, including protecting clients' right to privacy and confidentiality in the counseling/therapy relationship and the information resulting from it, and to notify clients that their right to privacy and confidentiality will not be violated by the supervisory relationship.

D. Records of the counseling/therapy relationship, including interview notes, test data, correspondence, the electronic storage of these documents, and audio and videotape recordings are considered to be confidential professional information. Supervisors shall assure that these materials are used in counseling/therapy, research, and training and supervision of counselors and therapists with the full knowledge of the client and that permission to use these materials is granted by the applied counseling setting offering service to the client. This professional information is to be used for the full protection of the client.

E. Written consent from the client (or legal guardian, if a minor) shall be secured prior to the use of such information for instructional, supervisory, and/or research purposes. Policies of the applied counseling setting regarding client records also shall be followed.

F. Supervisors shall adhere to current professional and legal guidelines when conducting research with human participants.

G. Supervisors are responsible for making every effort to monitor both professional actions , and failure to take action, of their supervisees.

16.3 Supervisory Role. The primary obligation of supervisors is to train counselors and therapists so that they respect the integrity and promote the welfare of the client. Inherent and integral to the role of supervisor are responsibilities for:

A. monitoring client welfare;

B. encouraging compliance with relevant legal, ethical and professional standards of clinical practice;

C. monitoring clinical performance and professional development of supervisees; and

D. evaluating and certifying current performance and potential of supervisee for academic, screening, selection, placement, employment, and credentialing purposes.

16.4 Supervisors should have had training and experience in supervision prior to initiating their role as supervisors.

16.5 Supervisors shall pursue professional and personal continuing education activities such as advanced courses, seminars, and professional conferences on a regular and on-going basis. These activities should include both counseling/ therapy and supervision topics and skills.

16.6 Supervisors shall inform their supervisee of professional and ethical standards and legal responsibilities of the counseling/therapy profession.

16.7 Supervisors of postgraduate counselors and therapists who are seeking state licensure should encourage these counselors and therapists to adhere to the standards of practice established by the state licensure board of the state in which they practice.

16.8 Procedures for contacting the supervisor, or an alternative supervisor, to assist in handling crisis situations shall be established and communicated to supervisees.

16.9 Actual work samples via session process notes, audio/videotape or live observation in addition to case notes shall be reviewed by the supervisor as a regular part of the ongoing supervisory process.

16.10 Supervisors shall meet regularly in face-to-face sessions with their supervisees.

16.11 Supervisors shall provide supervisees with ongoing feedback on their performance. This feedback should take a variety of forms, both formal and informal, and should include verbal and written evaluations. It should be formative during the supervisory experience and summative at the conclusion of the experience.

16.12 Supervisors who have multiple roles (e.g., teacher, clinical supervisor, administrative supervisor, etc.) with supervisees shall minimize potential conflicts. Where possible, the roles should be divided among several and it should be conveyed to the supervisee as to the expectations and responsibilities associated with each supervisory role.

16.13 Supervisors shall not participate in any form of sexual contact with supervisees. Dual relationships with supervisees that might impair the supervisor's objectivity and professional judgment should be avoided and/or the supervisory relationship terminated.

16.14 Supervisors shall not establish a psychotherapeutic relationship as a substitute for supervision. Personal issues should be addressed in supervision only in terms of the impact of these issues on clients and on professional functioning.

16.15 Supervisors, through ongoing supervisee assessment and evaluation, should be aware of any personal or professional limitations of supervisees which are likely to impede future professional performance. Supervisors have the responsibility of recommending remedial assistance to the supervisee and of screening from the training program, applied counseling setting, or state licensure those supervisees who are unable to provide competent professional services. These recommendations should be clearly and professionally explained in writing to the supervisees who are so evaluated.

16.16 Supervisors shall not endorse a supervisee for certification, licensure, completion of an academic training program, or continued employment if the supervisor believes the supervisee is impaired in any way that would interfere with the performance of counseling/therapy duties. The presence of any such impairment should begin the process of feedback and remediation wherever possible so that the supervisee understands the nature of the impairment and has the opportunity to remedy the problem and continue with his/her professional development.

16.17 Supervisors shall supervise clinical work only in areas where they are fully competent, and experienced.

16.18 Supervisors shall inform supervisees of the goals, policies, theoretical orientations towards counseling/therapy, training, and supervision model or approach on which supervision is based.

16.19 Supervisors shall use the following prioritized sequence in resolving conflicts among the needs of the client, the needs of the supervisee, and the needs of the program or the agency. Insofar as the client must be protected, it shall be understood that client welfare is usually subsumed in federal and state laws such that these statutes should be the first point of reference. Where laws and ethical standards are not present or are unclear, the good judgment of the supervisor shall be guided by the following list:
A. relevant legal and ethical standards (e.g., duty to warn, state child abuse laws, etc.);
B. client welfare;
C. supervisee welfare;
D. supervisor welfare;
E. program and/or agency service and administrative needs.

# REFERENCES

Alberding, B., Lauver, P., & Patnoe, J. (1993). Counselor awareness of the consequences of certification and licensure. *Journal of Counseling & Development, 72* (1), 33-38.

Aldridge, D. (1990). Toward a common language among the creative arts therapies. *The Arts in Psychotherapy, 17*, 189-196.

Allen, P. B. (1992). Artist-in-residence: An alternative to "clinification" for art therapists. *Art Therapy: Journal of the American Art Therapy Association, 9 (1),* 22-29.

American Art Therapy Association. (1987). Model job description. Mundelein, IL: Author. [This document can also be found in M. B. Junge with P. P. Asawa (1994), *A History of Art Therapy in the United States*, Mundelein, IL: AATA, Inc.]

American Art Therapy Association. (1992). *General standards of practice document.* Mundelein, IL: Author.

American Art Therapy Association. (1990). *Definition of art therapy assessment.* Mundelein, IL: Author.

American Art Therapy Association. (1992). *Bylaws.* Mundelein, IL: Author.

American Art Therapy Association. (1994). *Education Standards,* Mundelein, IL: Author.

American Art Therapy Association. (1995). *Ethical standards for art therapists (includes definition of independent practitioner).* Mundelein, IL: Author.

American Counseling Association. (1995). *Standards of practice and ethical standards.* Washington, DC: Author.

American Psychiatric Association. (1994). *Diagnostic and statistical manual of mental disorders (4th ed.).* Washington, DC: Author.

American Psychological Association (1991). *Guidelines for providers of psychological services to ethnic, linguistic, and culturally diverse populations.* Washington, DC. Author.

American Psychological Association (1994). *Publication manual of the American Psychological Association (4th ed.).* Washington, DC. Author.

American Psychological Association. (1993). *APA code of ethics.* Washington, DC: Author.

Amundson, N. E. (1988). The use of metaphor and drawings in case conceptualization. *Journal of Counseling and Development, 66*, 391-393.

Andersen, T. (1987). The reflecting team: Dialogue and meta-dialogue in clinical work. *Family Process, 26* (4), 415-428.

Anderson, H. & Goolishian, H. (1988). Human systems as linguistic systems:

Preliminary and evolving ideas about the implications for clinical theory. *Family Process, 27,* 371-394.

Ard, B. N. (1973). Providing clinical supervision for marriage counselors. A model for supervisor or supervisee. *The Family Coordinators, 22,*91-97.

Art Therapy Credentials Board (1996). *Bulletin of information.* Chicago, IL: Author.

Art Therapy Credentials Board (1996). *A.T.R. registration application.* Chicago, IL: Author.

Art Therapy Credentials Board. (1996). *Certification examination study guide.* Chicago, IL: Author.

Ault, R. (1977). Are you an artist or therapist—A professional dilemma of art therapists. In R. Shoemaker & S. Gonick-Barris (eds.), Creativity and the Art Therapist's Identity (pp. 53- 56), *Proceedings of the 7th Annual AATA Conference.* Baltimore, MD: AATA.

Austin, K., Moline, M., & Williams, G. (1990). *Confronting malpractice: Legal and ethical dilemmas in psychotherapy.* Newbury Park, CA: Sage.

Baker, B. (1994, July/August). Art therapy's growing pains. *Common Boundary,* 42-48.

Belfiore, M., & Cagnoletta, M.D. (1992). Arts therapy in Italy: Toward a pedagogical model. *The Arts in Psychotherapy, 19* (2) 111-116.

Bennett, B. Bryant, B., VandenBos, G., & Greenwood, A. (1990). *Professional liability and risk management.* Washington, DC: American Psychological Association.

Berger, M., & Dammann, C (1982). Live supervision as context, treatment, and training. *Family Process, 21* (3), 337-344.

Biggs, D. A. (1988). A case presentation approach in clinical supervision. *Counselor Education & Supervision, 27,* 240-248.

Borders, L. D. (1991). A systematic approach to peer group supervision. *Journal of Counseling & Development, 69,* 248-252.

Braverman, J. (1995). Retention of treatment records under the new AATA Ethics Standards. *AATA Newsletter, XXVII* (1), 15.

California Association of Marriage and Family Therapists. (1990). *Practical applications in supervision: A manual for supervisors.* San Diego, CA: Author.

Calisch, A. (1989). Eclectic blending of theory in the supervision of art psychotherapists. *The Arts in Psychotherapy, 16,* 37-43.

Carifio, M. S., & Hess, A. K. (1987). Who is the ideal supervisor? *Professional psychology: Research and Practice, 3,* 244-250.

Carrigan, J. (1993). Ethical considerations in a supervisory relationship: A synthesis. *Art Therapy: Journal of the American Art Therapy Association, 10* (3), 130-135.

Cattaneo, M. (1994). Addressing culture and values in the training of art therapists. *Art Therapy: Journal of the American Art Therapy Association, 11*(3), 184-186.

Cattaneo, M., & Gawalek, M. (1994). Ethical guidelines for core and adjunct faculty: Multiple roles. *Unpublished guidelines from Lesley College Counseling and Expressive Therapies Division.*

Charney, I. W. (1986). What do therapists worry about? A tool for experiential supervision. In F. Kaslow (ed.), *Supervision and Training.* (p. 17-28). New York: Haworth Press.

Cohen, B. & Cox, C. (1995). *Telling without talking.* New York: W. W. Norton.

Cohen, M., Gross, S. & Turner, M. (1976). A note on a developmental model for training family therapists through group supervision. *Journal of Marriage and Family Counseling, 2,* 48-56.

Cohen-Lieberman, M. S. (1994). The art therapist as expert witness in child sexual abuse. *Art Therapy: The Journal of the American Art Therapy Association. 11* (4) 260-265.

Colapinto, J. (1988). Teaching the structural way, In H. Liddle, H., D. Bruelin, & R. Schwartz (Eds.), *Handbook of Family Therapy Training and Supervision* (p. 17-37). New York: The Guilford Press.

Committee on Lesbian and Gay Concerns. (1991). Avoiding heterosexual bias in language. *American Psychologist, 46* (9), 973-974.

Corey , G., & Corey, M. (1990). Learning to wrestle with ethical dilemmas, *Guidepost, 18,* 24.

Corey, G., Corey, M.S., & Callanan, P. (1993). *Issues and ethics in the helping professions:* Pacific Grove, CA: Brooks/Cole.

Cox, L. (1990). Integrative evaluations: Some processed oriented questions for supervisors. In *Practical Applications in Supervision* (pp. 85-90). San Diego: CAMFT.

Deegan, P. (1993). Recovering our sense of value after being labeled. *Journal of Psychiatric Nursing, 31* (4), 7-11.

Doehrman, M. J. G. (1976). Parallel process in supervision and psychotherapy. *Bulletin of Menninger Clinic., 40*(1),103-104.

Dufrene, P. (1991). Comparison of treatment of traditional education of native American healers with education of American art therapists. *Art Therapy: Journal of the American Art Therapy Association, 8 (1),* 17-22.

Dulcai, D. (1984). The challenge we face. *The Arts in Psychotherapy, 11,* 247-248.

Dulicai, C., Hays, R. , & Nolan, P. (1989). Training the creative arts therapist: Identity with integration. *The Arts in Psychotherapy, 16*(1),11-14.

277

Durkin, J., Perach, D., Ramseyer, J., & Sontag, E. (1989). A model for art therapy supervision enhanced through art making and journal writing. In H. Wadeson, J. Durkin, & D. Perach (Eds.), *Advances in Art Therapy* (pp. 390-431). New York: Wiley.

Dye, H. A., & Borders, L. D. (1990). Counseling supervisors: Standards for preparation and practice. *Journal of Counseling & Development, 69,* 27-32.

Edwards, D. (1993). Learning about feelings: The role of supervision in art therapy training. *The Arts in Psychotherapy, 20,* 213-222.

Edwards, D. (1994). On reflection: A note on supervision. *Inscape, 1* (1), 23-27.

Ekstein, R., & Wallerstein, R. (1972). *The teaching and learning of psychotherapy.* New York. Basic Books.

Ellis, M. V., & Douce, L. A. (1994). Group supervision of novice clinical supervisors: Eight recurring issues. *Journal of Counseling & Development, 72,* 520-525.

Fineberg, M. (1993). Training art therapy students to be supervisors: ethical and practical issues. *American Journal of Art Therapy, 31*(2),.109-112.

Fisch, R. (1988). Training in the brief therapy model. In H. Liddle, H., D. Bruelin, & R. Schwartz (Eds.), *Handbook of Family Therapy Training and Supervision.* (p. 78-92). New York: The Guilford Press.

Fish, B. (1989). Addressing countertransference through image making. In H. Wadeson, J. Durkin, & D. Perach (Eds.), *Advances in Art Therapy* (pp. 376-389). New York: Wiley.

Frantz, T. G. (1990). Developmental stages in supervision: Implications for supervisors and administrators. In *CAMFT Manual for Supervisors.* (p. 3-8-22). San Diego, CA: CAMFT.

Freeny, M. (1994). Getting well in the fast lane. *Family Therapy Networker, 18*(2), 73-76.

Friedman, D., & Kaslow, J. N. (1986). The development of professional identity in psychotherapists: Six stages in the supervision process. In F. W. Kaslow (ed.), *Supervision and Training: Models, Dilemmas, and Challenges.* (p.29-50). New York: Haworth Press.

Gardner, H. (1984). *Artful scribbles.* New York: Basic Books.

Gardner, M. H. (1980). Racial, ethnic and social class considerations in psychotherapy supervision. In, A. K. Hess (ed.), *Psychotherapy.* ( p. 474-508). New York: Wiley & Sons.

Gergen, K. (1991). *The saturated self: Dilemmas of identity in contemporary life.* New York: Basic Books.

Gillen, J. S. (1990). Different types of countertransference and the importance of addressing them in supervision. In *CAMFT Manual for Supervisors.* (p. 3-156-160). San Diego, CA: CAMFT.

Gilligan, C. (1982). *In a different voice.* Cambridge, MA: Harvard University Press.

Goldenberg, I., & Goldenberg, H. (1991). *Family therapy: An overview.* Pacific Grove, CA: Brooks/Cole Publishers.

Goldenthal, P. (1993). A matter of balance: Challenging and supporting supervisees. *The Supervision Bulletin (AAMFT), 3* (2), 1-2.

Good, D. (1993). The history of art therapy licensure in New Mexico. *Art Therapy: Journal of the American Art Therapy Association, 10*(3), 136-140.

Haley, J. (1976). *Problem solving therapy* .San Francisco: Jossey-Bass.

Haley, J. (1976). Problems of training therapists. In J. Haley (Ed.) *Problem-Solving Therapy* (pp. 169-194). San Francisco. Jossey-Bass.

Haley, J. (1988). Reflections on therapy supervision. In H. Liddle, D. Breulin, & R. Schwartz (Eds.), *Handbook of Family and Marital Therapy* (pp. 358-367). New York. Guilford Press.

Hare-Mustin, R. (1976). Live supervision in psychotherapy. *Voices, 12,* 21-24.

Hawkins, P. & Shoret, R. (1989). *Supervision in the helping professions.* Open University Press.

Hess, A. K. (1980). *Psychotherapy supervision: Theory, research and practice.* New York: Wiley & Sons.

Hillman, J., & Ventura, M. (1993). *We've had a hundred years of psychotherapy—and the world's getting worse.* San Francisco: HarperSanFrancisco.

Hines, M. (1993). In my opinion: Dual aspects of dual relationships. *The Supervision Bulletin (AAMFT), 6* (3), 3.

Hoffman, L. (1993). *Exchanging voices.* London: H. Karnac.

Holloway, E. (1995). *Clinical supervision: A systems approach.* Thousand Oaks, CA: Sage.

Holloway, E. L., & Johnston, R. (1985). Group supervision: Widely practiced but poorly understood. *Counselor Education & Supervision, 24,* 332-340.

Holloway, E. L. (1994). Overseeing the overseer: Contextualizing training in supervision. *Journal of Counseling & Development, 72,* 526-530.

Howie, P., & Gutierrez, K. G. (1994). *The continuous quality improvement manual.* Mundelein, IL: AATA, Inc.

Irwin, E. C. (1986). On being and becoming a therapist. *The Arts in Psychotherapy, 13,* 191-195.

Ishiyama, F. I. (1988). A model of visual case processing using metaphors and drawings. *Counselor Education & Supervision, 28,* 153-161.

Jenerson. D. S. (1990). Practical and cultural aspects of supervision. In *Practical Applications in Supervision* (pp. 43-51). San Diego: CAMFT.

Johnson, D. (1984). Establishing the creative arts therapies as an independent profession. *The Arts in Psychotherapy, 11,* 209-212.

Johnson, D. (1985). Envisioning the link among the creative arts therapies, *The Arts In Psychotherapy, 12*, 233-238.

Junge, M. (1989). Co-perspective: The heart of the matter. *The Arts in Psychotherapy, 16* (2), 77-78.

Junge, M., Alvarez, J. F., Kellogg, A., & Volker, C. (1993). The art therapist as social activist. *Art Therapy: Journal of the American Art Therapy Association, 10*(3), 148-155.

Kalichman, S.C. (1993). *Mandated reporting of suspected child abuse.* Washington, DC: American Psychological Association.

Kaslow, F. (1977). *Supervision, consultation and staff training in the helping professions.* San Francisco: Jossey-Bass.

Knapp, J., Knapp, L., & Phillips, J. (1994). Report on the national art therapy practice analysis survey. *Art Therapy: Journal of the American Art Therapy Association, 11*(2), 146-150.

Lawless, M. (1995). *The Family Therapy Networker,* Vol. 19, #4, p. 24.

Lachman-Chapin, M. (1993). The art therapist as exhibiting artist. *Art Therapy: Journal of the American Art Therapy Association, 10*(3), 141-147.

Levick, M., Safran, D., & Levine, A. (1990). Art therapists as expert witnesses: A judge delivers a precedent-setting decision. *The Arts in Psychotherapy, 17*, 49-53.

Levenson, P. (1986). Identification of child abuse in art and play products of pediatric burn patients. *Art Therapy; Journal of the American Art Therapy Association, 3* (2).

Liddel, H.,& Saba, G. (1982). Teaching family therapy at the introductory level: A model emphasizing a pattern which connects training and therapy. *Journal of Marital & Family Therapy, 8*, 63-72.

Liddle, H., Breulin, D., Schwartz, R. & Constantine, J. (1984). Training family therapy supervisors: Issues of content, form and context. *Journal of Marital & Family Therapy. 10*, 139-150.

Lipchik, E. (1994). The rush to be brief. *Family Therapy Networker, 18* (2), 34-39.

Lippin, R. A. (1985). Arts medicine. *The Arts in Psychotherapy, 12*, 147-49.

Malchiodi, C. (1990). *Breaking the silence: Art therapy with children from violent homes.* New York: Brunner/Mazel.

Malchiodi, C. A, (1994). Introduction to special section on assessment. *Art Therapy: Journal of the American Art Therapy Association, 11*(1), 104.

Malchiodi, C. A. (1991). Using drawings in the evaluation of children from violent homes. *Family Violence & Sexual Assault Bulletin, 7* (4), 14-16.

Malchiodi, C. A. (1992). Writing for publication. *Art Therapy: Journal of the American Art Therapy Association, 9* (2), 62- 64.

Malchiodi, C. A. (1993). Is there a crisis in art therapy education? *Art Therapy: Journal of the American Art Therapy Association, 10* (3).

Malchiodi, C. A. (1993). Medical art therapy: Defining the field. *International Journal of Arts Medicine, 2* (1).

Malchiodi, C. A. (1994). Certification: In search of accountability. *Art Therapy: Journal of the American Art Therapy Association, 11* (3), 170-172.

Malchiodi, C. A. (1994). Family art therapy and postmodern society. In Riley, S. with C. Malchiodi, *Integrative Approaches to Family Art Therapy* (pp. 213-221). Chicago: Magnolia Street.

Malchiodi, C. A. (1994). Sorting out certification. *Art Therapy: Journal of the American Art Therapy Association, 11*(2), 82-83.

Malchiodi, C. A. (1995). Who owns the art ? *Art Therapy: Journal of the American Art Therapy Association, 12* (1), 2-3.

Malchiodi, C. A., Allen, P. B., & Cattaneo, M. (1991). Art therapy: Postmortem. *Opening session presentation at the Annual AATA Conference*, Denver, CO. National Audio Video #1-135 [ 4465 Washington Avenue, Denver, CO 80216].

McGoldrick, M., & Gerson, R. (1987). *Genograms in family assessment.* New York: Norton.

McGoldrick, M., Anderson, C., & Walsh, F. (1989). *Women in families: A framework for family therapy.* New York: W. W. Norton.

McKim, R. H. (1972). *Experiences in visual thinking.* Monterey, CA: Brooks/ Cole.

McNiff, S. (1986). *Educating the creative arts therapist.* Springfield, IL: Charles C Thomas.

McNiff, S. (1991). Ethics and the autonomy of images. *The Arts in Psychotherapy, 18,* 277-283.

Meriwether, M. H. (1986). Child abuse reporting laws: Time for a change. *Family Law Quarterly, 20,* 141-174.

Molvado, B. (1992). Live supervision as a window. *The American Association of Marriage & Family Therapy Supervision Bulletin, 5* (2), 1-2.

Moon, C. (1994). What's been left behind: The place of the art product in art therapy. In *Proceedings of the 25th Annual AATA Conference* (p.108), Mundelein, IL: AATA, Inc.

New Mexico Counseling and Therapy Board. (1993). *Counselor and therapist practice act.* Santa Fe, NM: Author.

Nichols, M. P., & Schwartz, R. C. (1995). *Family therapy: Concepts and methods.* Boston, MA: Boston, Allyn and Bacon.

Nichols, W. (1988). Family therapy/education training: An integrative psychodynamic and systems approach. In. H. A. Liddle, D.C. Breulin, &

R. C. Schwartz (eds.) *Handbook of family therapy training and supervision.* (p. 110-127). New York: Guilford.

O'Hara, M., & Anderson, W. T. (1991, September/October). Welcome to the postmodern world. *Family Therapy Networker,* 19-25.

Papp, P. (1980). The Greek chorus and other techniques of paradoxical therapy, *Family Process, 19,*45-57

Parsons, P. (1986). Outsider art: Patient art enters the art world. *American Journal of Art Therapy, 25,* 3-12.

Pirotta, S, & Cecchin, G. (1988). The Milan training program. In H. Liddle, H., D. Bruelin, & R. Schwartz (Eds.), *Handbook of Family Therapy Training and Supervision* (p. 38-61). New York: The Guilford Press.

Pope, K. S., & Vasquez, M. (1991). *Ethics in psychotherapy and counseling: A practical guide for psychologists.* San Francisco: Jossey-Bass.

Rabin, M. (1993). Full circle. *Art Therapy: Journal of the American Art Therapy Association, 10,* 171-172.

Research and Training Center on Independent Living. (1993). *Guidelines for reporting and writing about people with disabilities (3rd. ed.).* Lawrence, KS: University of Kansas.

Riley, S. (1994). Art therapy in the 21st century. *Art Therapy: Journal of the American Art Therapy Association, 11*(2), 100-101.

Riley, S. (1994). Change: The reality of the mental health providers' world in the 1990's. In Riley, S. &. C. Malchiodi, *Integrative Approaches to Family Art Therapy* (pp. 247-256). Chicago: Magnolia Street.

Riley, S., & Malchiodi, C. (1994). *Integrative approaches to family art therapy.* Chicago: Magnolia Street Press.

Rinas, J., & Clyne-Jackson, S. (1988). *Professional conduct and legal concerns in mental health practice.* San Mateo, CA: Appleton & Lange.

Robbins, A. (1988). A psychoaesthetic perspective on creative arts therapy and training. *The Arts in Psychotherapy, 15* (4),95-100.

Rogers, C. (1957). Training individuals to engage in the therapeutic process. In C. R. Strother (Ed.), *Psychology and Mental Health* (pp. 72-96). Washington, DC: American Psychological Association.

Roth, S. (1986). Peer supervision in the community mental health center: An analysis and critique. *The Clinical Supervisor, 4,* 159-168.

Rubin, J. (1984). *The art of art therapy.* New York: Brunner/Mazel.

Runkel, T, & Hackney, H. (1982). Counselor peer supervision: A model and a challenge. *The Personnel and Guidance Journal, 61,* 113-115.

Ryder, R., & Hepworth, J. (1990). AAMFT ethical code: "Dual relationships." *Journal of Marital & Family Therapy, 16* (2), 127-132.

Sandel, S. (1989). On being a female creative arts therapist. *The Arts in*

*Psychotherapy, 16*, 239-242.

Schwartz, R. (1987). The trainer-trainee relationship in family therapy training. In. H. A. Liddle, D.C. Breulin, & R. C. Schwartz (eds.) *Handbook of Family Therapy and Supervision.* (p. 172-182). New York: Guilford Press.

Sluzki, C. (1974). Treatment, training, and research. Unpublished paper presented at the *Ackerman Memorial Conference* in Venezuela.

Sluzki, C. (1979). Migration and family conflict. *Family Process, 18*, 379-390.

Smart, M. (1986). Expanded work settings. *Art Therapy: Journal of the American Art Therapy Association, 3*, 21-26.

Spaniol, S. (1990a). Exhibiting art by people with mental illness: Issues, process and principles. *Art Therapy: Journal of the American Art Therapy Association, 2*, 70-78.

Spaniol, S. (1990b). *Organizing exhibitions of art by people with mental illness: A step-by-step manual.* Boston: Center for Psychiatric Rehabilitation, Boston University.

Spaniol, S. (1994). Confidentiality reexamined: Negotiating use of art by clients. *American Journal of Art Therapy, 32* (3), 69- 74.

Spaniol, S., & Cattaneo, M. (1994). The power of language in the art therapeutic relationship. *Art Therapy, Journal of the American Art Therapy Association, 11* (4) 266-270.

Spice, C., & Spice, W. (1976). A triadic method of supervision in the training of counselors and counseling supervisors. *Counselor Education & Supervision, 15*, 251-258.

Spring, D. (1993). *Shattered images: Phenomonological language of sexual trauma.* Chicago, IL: Magnolia Street Publishers.

Steinhart, L. (1986). Art therapy in Israel. *Art Therapy, Journal of the American Art Therapy Association, 1* (3), 3-6.

Steiny, N. (1995). Editorial. *Newsletter: California Association of Marriage & Family Therapists, 1*, 2.

Tarasoff v. Regents of the University of California, 113 Cal. Rptr. 14, 551, P.2D.334. (Cal. 1976).

Tarasoff v. Regents of the University of California, 118 Cal. Rptr. 129, 529 P.2D.533. (Cal. 1974).

Vandecreek, L., & Knapp, S. (1984). Counselors, confidentiality, and life-endangering clients. *Counselor Education & Supervision*, 51-57.

Wadeson, H. (1994). Question: Will art therapy survive universal health coverage reform? *Art Therapy: Journal of the American Art Therapy Association, 11* (1), 26-28.

Wadeson, H. (Ed.)(1992). *A guide to conducting art therapy research.* Mundelein,

IL: AATA, Inc.

Wagner, C., & Smith, J. (1979). Peer supervision: Toward more effective training. *Counselor Education & Supervision, 18*, 288-293.

Webster, M. (1994). Legal and ethical issues impacting unlicensed art therapists and their clients in California. *Art Therapy: Journal of the American Art Therapy Association, 11* (4), 278-281.

Weinrach, S., & Thomas, K. R. (1993). The National Board for Certifying Counselors (NBCC): The good, the bad and the ugly. *Journal of Counseling & Development, 72* (1), 105-109.

Whiffen, R. (1982). *The use of videotape in supervision: Recent developments in practice.* London: Academic Press.

Whitaker, C. (1976). Comment: Live supervision in psychotherapy. *Voices, 12,* 24-25.

Whitaker, C. (1989). *Midnight musings of a family therapist.* New York: W.W. Norton & Company.

White, M. (1994). Panning for gold. *The Family Therapy Networker, 18* (6), 40-49.

White, M. & Epston, D. (1990). *Narrative means to therapeutic ends.* New York: W.W. Norton & Co.

Wilson, L. (1987). Confidentiality in art therapy: An ethical dilemma. *American Journal of Art Therapy, 25,* 75-80.

Wilson, L., Riley, S., & Wadeson, H. (1984). Art therapy supervision. *Art Therapy: Journal of the American Art Therapy Association, 1* (3), 100-105.

Wilson, S. (1981). *Field instruction: Techniques for supervisors.* London: Macmillan.

Wirtz, G. (1994). Essential legal issues for art therapists in private practice. *Art Therapy: Journal of the American Art Therapy Association, 11* (4), 293-296.

Wirtz, G., Sidun, N., Carrigan, J., Wadeson, H., Kennedy, S., & Marano-Geiser, R. (1994). *Legal issues: Can art therapists stand alone?* Denver, CO: National Audio Video tape # 58-149.

Wix, L. (1995). The Intern Studio: A pilot study. *Art Therapy: Journal of the American Art Therapy Association, 12*(3), 175-178.

Wolber, G., & Carne, W. (1993). *Writing psychological reports.* Sarasota, FL: Professional Resource Press.

Wylie, M.S. (1994). Endangered species. *Family Therapy Networker, 18* (2), 20-33.

Zuckerman, E. (1995). *Clinician's thesaurus: The guidebook for writing psychological reports.* New York: The Guilford Press.

# Cathy A. Malchiodi, MA, A.T.R., LPAT, LPCC

Cathy A. Malchiodi is a graduate of the Boston Museum School/Tufts University and the College of Notre Dame and is a licensed professional art therapist and licensed professional clinical counselor. She is widely published in the field of art therapy, serving as the current Editor of *Art Therapy: Journal of the American Art Therapy Association* and is the author of more than 40 refereed publications, particularly on the use of art expression with trauma victims, dissociative disorders, child physical and sexual abuse, domestic violence, physical illness, and arts medicine. She is the author of *Breaking the Silence: Art Therapy with Children from Violent Homes* (Brunner/Mazel, 1990; revised edition 1996), co-author of *Integrative Approaches to Family Art Therapy* (Magnolia Street Publishers, 1994), and recently completed a chapter on art therapy with women with breast cancer for the forthcoming book *Women and Art Therapy: Visions of Difference.* She currently serves on the Editorial Boards of the *International Journal of Arts Medicine, Journal of Child Sexual Abuse,* and the *Journal of Alternative Medicine.*

Ms. Malchiodi has also been featured in a variety of media, including videos produced by the Kennedy Center, China Central Television (CCTV), the Breast Cancer Action Group, and various training videos for therapists and clinicians, and in articles including *Very Special Arts International Magazine,* the *Boston Globe,* and various releases by the Associated Press. In December 1995 she was interviewed on both the British Broadcasting Company (BBC) and Tokyo Today on her work using art therapy with medical populations and as a form of alternative medicine. She has been a consultant to clinical, educational and corporate organizations including universities throughout the US and abroad, a variety of clinics, hospitals and community agencies, and organizations such as the Educational Testing Service (ETS) in Princeton, BRAVO Network, Sage Publications, Very Special Arts, and WGBN/Public Broadcasting Station, among others.

Active in the profession of art therapy, Cathy was elected to the Executive Board of the American Art Therapy Association (AATA) for four years, serving as Secretary and a member of the Executive Committee, and has been appointed chair of various AATA committees, including Membership, Ethics, Certification, and Publications. She has received numerous awards for her work in art therapy including special awards from China Fund for the Handicapped, the Hong Kong Department of Social Services, and the US Information Agency; Outstanding Educator Award, Very Special Arts; the Art Therapy Pioneer Award; the Thomas Dee Fellowship for Teaching and Research; and in 1991 she received the Distinguished Service Award for her work with the American Art Therapy Association and contributions to the field of art therapy.

Ms. Malchiodi has an international reputation as an educator and has been a visiting professor at universities, colleges, and institutions throughout the US, Canada, Europe, and Asia. She has given over 100 invited presentations on the topic of art therapy, nationally and internationally. She has worked as a Master Teacher for Very Special Arts International and was selected in 1987 to represent them in China, the first educational exchange of its kind and led the first Very Special Arts Festival Beijing, China, at the United States Embassy. Cathy also served as the Interim Director of the Art Therapy/ Marriage and Family Counseling Degree program at California State University, Sacramento, and also as the former Director of the Art Therapy Graduate Program at the University of Utah. She is currently on the adjunct faculty of Lesley College, Expressive Therapies Department, and Southwestern College, and is the Director of the Institute for the Arts & Health, a national training and research institute devoted to the development of the expressive arts as an adjunct to a total wellness program.

Cathy has served as an expert witness in legal cases, particularly those involving the use of drawings to identify physical and sexual abuse and her private practice and consultation services specialize in forensic and medical art therapy with children, adults, and families. Currently, she is investigating the role of art making and writing in the comprehensive medical care of individuals with breast cancer, AIDS/HIV, and other illnesses. In addition to her work as an art therapist, Cathy is an active visual artist, exhibiting paintings, mixed media and assemblages in regional and national shows. She is married to David F. Barker, a research scientist and human geneticist, and currently lives in Salt Lake City, UT.

## Shirley Riley, MA, A.T.R., MFCT

Shirley Riley has been a Registered Art Therapist since 1976 and a licensed Marriage and Family Counselor, California, since 1979. She is an Approved AAMFT Supervisor and conducts a private practice in West Los Angeles where she sees families, couples and individuals and supervises interns and colleagues.

As Adjunct Associate Professor for Loyola Marymount University's Marital and Family Art Therapy graduate program, Ms. Riley teaches Advanced Family Art Therapy and has been the Placement Coordinator until this year, 1996. In that capacity she has been responsible for the supervision of supervisors as well as students. She held the position of Associate Chair of the department for a year; taught a variety of courses, including Group Dynamics, Adolescent Developmental Art Therapy and Multicultural Issues. In addition, she holds an adjunct professorship position at Pepperdine University, Los Angeles, teaching Family Therapy and Practicum Supervision. As an expert in her field she is regularly invited to lecture at universities and Professional Institutions in the United States, the Netherlands, Canada, Australia and Japan.

Ms. Riley received the Outstanding Clinician Award from the American Association of Art Therapy in 1990. Her book *Integrative Approaches to Family Art Therapy*, Magnolia Street Publishers, Chicago, IL was published in 1994. Her clinical work has been published in journals and edited books, both in and outside the field of art therapy.

Shirley Riley served on the Board of Directors of the American Art Therapy Association for six years, has been on the Education Committee and the Education and Training Board and is presently Chair of the Long Range

Planning Committee and a member of the editorial board of *Art Therapy: Journal of the American Art Therapy Association.*

In her personal life she has been most fortunate to have been supported and encouraged by her husband, her four sons and their wives, and eight grandchildren. Her husband's profession as an MD provided a background of ethics and caring that inspired her choice of career.

# Magnolia Street Publishers

**Supervision and Related Issues: A Handbook for Professionals    *MALCHIODI & RILEY***
A highly informative guide to the complexities of supervision in the 90's. Supervisors, educators, and students will find it indispensable in their sessions, the classroom and in work with clients. An extensive appendix includes ethics and standards of practice, sample forms for use in supervision, laws effecting supervisors and many more references and resources. (300 pages)

**The Gestalt Art Experience: Patterns That Connect                *JANIE RHYNE***
Based on gestalt psychology and therapy, the focus of this book is on direct and immediate experiential insights gained through creating art that expresses and clarifies personal problems and potential. Emphasis is on exploring present life style and discovering possibilities for self-actualization. (revised edition, color illustrations, 225 pages)

**Art Therapy in Theory & Practice                *ed. ELINOR ULMAN & P. DACHINGER***
Since its first publication, this volume has been used continually as both a textbook and a resource. Many of the chapters have become indispensable classics which continue to define the field of art therapy. Elinor Ulman shows great skill, perception and eloquence as both a writer and editor. (color illustrations, 414 pages)

**Integrative Approaches To Family Art Therapy  *SHIRLEY RILEY & CATHY MALCHIODI***
This important new book by noted family art therapist Shirley Riley is designed for both the beginning practitioner as well as the advanced family therapist. An important source of ideas, this text provides not only examples of integrative approaches to family art therapy, but also offers practical ways to utilize art therapy with individuals, families and couples. Chapters cover a wide range of theoretical viewpoints, including structural, systemic, narrative, family of origin and social constructionism. (262 pages)

**Art As Therapy With Children                *EDITH KRAMER***
Kramer's discussions of sublimation, art and defense, aggression, and the role of the art therapist have not been surpassed by later volumes or by other authors. This profoundly wise volume offers inspiration and genuine assistance to the fledgling clinician as well as to anyone else working with children who wishes to understand how and why art can have such a profound effect. (color illustrations,238 pages)

**Shattered Images: Phenomenological Language of Sexual Trauma        *DEE SPRING***
Dee Spring has specialized in the treatment of post-traumatic stress and dissociative disorders for more than twenty years. Her pioneering efforts in this field have gained international recognition because of her unique treatment style which includes art therapy, imagery and hypnosis. She presents a treatment model that simultaneously helps the therapist stay on track amid the myriad crises encountered with sexual trauma victims and creatively explains the complex, multi-level treatment process. (305 pages)

**Dynamically Oriented Art Therapy: It's Principles & Practice  *MARGARET NAUMBURG***
As a pioneer in this field of psychotherapy, Margaret Naumburg's approach to art therapy is psychoanalytically oriented; she recognized the fundamental importance of the unconscious as expressed in the patient's dreams, daydreams and fantasies. In this work, three case histories of emotionally disturbed women are used to illustrate the various ways in which the process of dynamically oriented art therapy can function in the treatment of depression, ulcers and alcoholism. (color illustrations,168 pages)

*5804 N. Magnolia St., Chicago, IL 60660,  312-561-2121, fax 312-477-6096*